Highest Yoga Tantra

An Introduction to the Esoteric Buddhism of Tibet

Highest Yoga Tantra

An Introduction to the Esoteric Buddhism of Tibet

Daniel Cozort

Snow Lion Publications
Ithaca, New York USA

Snow Lion Publications
P.O. Box 6483
Ithaca, New York 14851
USA

First Edition U.S.A. 1986

Printed in USA.

Library of Congress Catalogue Number 86–3800

ISBN 0–937938–32–7

Library of Congress Cataloging-in-Publication Data

Cozort, Daniel G., 1953–
    Highest yoga tantra.

    Includes bibliographies and index.
    1. Yoga (Tantric Buddhism)   I. Title.
BQ8938.C69   1986   294.3'925   86–3800
ISBN 0–937938–32–7

Contents

Charts

The drawings on pages 40 and 116 are by Sidney Piburn.

Technical Note

It is hoped that this book will be of use to the general reader as well as to Buddhologists who work with Tibetan and/or Sanskrit texts. For the latter, Tibetan and Sanskrit equivalents of key terms are furnished in an English-Sanskrit-Tibetan glossary. Transliteration has followed the system devised by Turrell Wylie.[1] Some key items in the glossary are marked with an asterisk upon their first occurrence.

For non-specialists, three procedures have been followed in the body of this book to increase its accessibility:

(1) Sanskrit and Tibetan words have been limited to parenthetical citation with two exceptions: a small number of Sanskrit terms are treated as English words, and proper names are not translated, except for book titles, which have been translated as an aid to understanding the contents of the books cited. The Sanskrit terms treated as English words, unencumbered by italicizing and diacritical marks, are: Bodhisattva, Buddha, karma, mandala, sutra, tantra, and yogi.

(2) Technical information deemed of interest but not of central importance has been placed in notes.

(3) A system of "essay phoenetics" that renders Tibetan and Sanskrit names in an easily pronounceable form, minus

marks for high tones, is used throughout the body of the book. It was devised by Professor Jeffrey Hopkins of the University of Virginia and is fully explained on pages 19 through 22 of his *Meditation on Emptiness* (London: Wisdom Publications, 1983). It is used because I share Professor Hopkins' feeling that mere transliteration places unnecessary obstacles in front of the reader who is not familiar with Tibetan and/or Sanskrit. For instance, it seems clear that no one whose native language is English could reasonably guess how to pronounce lcang-skya or 'jam-dbyangs-bzhad-pa. Names such as these are fated to remain alien and forgettable and may just as well have been reproduced in Tibetan script. Jang-gya and Jam-yang-shay-ba, on the other hand, are easy to pronounce and are easy to remember.

The problem with Sanskrit names is less acute. Still, because English speakers would tend to pronounce the first letter of Cakrasaṃvara as a hard *c* as in can rather than as *ch* as in chair, *ch* is used for *c*, resulting in Chakrasaṃvara; and because they would tend to pronounce the first letter of Śāntideva or the *ṣ* of Aśvaghoṣa as *s* as in so rather than, more correctly, as *sh* as in show, *sh* is used for *ś* and *ṣh* for *ṣ*, resulting in Shāntideva and Ashvaghoṣha. (*Chh* is used for *ch*.) Hyphens are placed between the syllables of Tibetan names not to reflect the fact that Tibetan itself punctuates each syllable by a dot, but to avert the incidence of confusing combinations such as Janggya or Tupdenngawang.

Acknowledgements

The greatest thanks must go to Professor Jeffrey Hopkins of the University of Virginia, for his wise and compassionate guidance through the complexities of Buddhist tantra. All of the preliminary work of translating Nga-wang-belden's the *Illumination of the Texts of Tantra* was completed under his direct supervision in a year-long class in 1980–81, which included Craig Preston, Jules Levinson, Katherine Rogers, Guy Newland, Leah Zahler, and Elizabeth Napper. Professor Hopkins brought all of his vast expertise to the class, correcting our sometimes miserable attempts at translation, conveying a great deal of information from his own extensive reading and from his long association with eminent Tibetan scholars, and stimulating us with his own critical insights. He has seen the present effort through several stages, at each point painstakingly identifying errors and ambiguities, and suggesting a multitude of ways to improve phrasing and structure. All of the virtues of this book may be traced to him; the defects I claim as my own.

I would also like to thank Professors Karen Christina Lang and M. Jamie Ferriera of the University of Virginia, Professor Donald S. Lopez of Middlebury College, and my wife, Christine Cozort, for reading and making helpful comments on the manuscript at various stages.

Preface

In the treasure-house of Tibetan Buddhism, tantra* is the
crown and Highest Yoga Tantra*[2] is its jewel. Greatest of
the four sets of tantras, the four collections of the Buddha's
secret discourses on practices intended for superior adepts,[3]
Highest Yoga Tantra is universally praised in Tibet as the
Buddha's most profound and wonderful teaching, granting
the most proficient of its practitioners the ability to reach
the ultimate rank of Buddhahood within just a single lifetime.

Like the Great Vehicle (*mahāyāna*) sutras*, the tantras
are traditionally considered to have been hidden after their
initial promulgation by the Buddha, not again emerging
into widespread practice until centuries later. Western
scholarship tends to assume that the tantras were actually
fabricated by Great Vehicle monks. In either case, the
earliest appearance of a tantra of the Highest Yoga Tantra
class is probably that of the *Guhyasamāja Tantra*, which can
be dated to the sixth century C. E. The Buddhist historian
Tāranātha reports that the other principal Highest Yoga
Tantras were procured by a series of teachers who lived
between 800 and 1040 C. E., the period of greatest tantric
activity in India.[4] This period roughly corresponds to the

era in which Buddhism was transmitted to Tibet, undoubtedly an important factor contributing to the high regard felt for tantra in Tibet. All of the schools of Tibetan Buddhism acknowledge the importance of tantra; initiation into the tantras and practice of them has been and continues to be a major part of the lives of Tibetan Buddhist adepts.

The main purpose of this book is to provide a map for the difficult terrain of Highest Yoga Tantra theory and practice. To that end, it identifies the prerequisites, stages, and sub-stages of Highest Yoga Tantra practice, explains technical tantric vocabulary, and explores several differences between two of the most important Highest Yoga tantras, the *Guhyasamāja Tantra* and the *Kālachakra Tantra*.

The presentation of Highest Yoga Tantra contained herein is based on an extraordinarily lucid Tibetan text concerned with the levels of attainment, or "grounds"* and "paths"*, of Highest Yoga Tantra. For the most part a presentation of the two stages of practice of the *Guhyasamāja Tantra*, the principal tantra of the Tibetan Ge-luk-ba (*dge lugs pa*) tradition,[5] it is entitled the *Illumination of the Texts of Tantra, Presentation of the Grounds and Paths of the Four Great Secret Tantra Sets.*[6] Its author, the nineteenth century Mongolian Ge-luk-ba scholar Nga-wang-bel-den (*ngag dbang dpal ldan*), is also noted for his many works on topics such as the Middle Way School*, the Perfection of Wisdom* literature, ultimate and conventional truths* in the four systems of Indian Buddhist tenets, and his annotations for Jam-yang-shay-ba's (*'jam dbyangs bzhad pa*) *Great Exposition of Tenets.*[7] The *Illumination of the Texts of Tantra* emphasizes the integral structure of Highest Yoga Tantra; it does not contain detailed descriptions of the initiations, permissions, visualized entities, and ritual acts that would be required for the actual practice of a tantra. Therefore, the present book also is mainly an outline or overview of the structure of Highest Yoga Tantra and is not meant to be a sufficient guide to its practice.

In this book, several sources have been utilized to clarify

and supplement the basic exposition of Highest Yoga Tantra found in the *Illumination of the Texts of Tantra*. Throughout the book, whenever any of these supplementary sources are used for clarification or contrast, they are footnoted; Nga-wang-bel-den's text itself, the basis for all of Parts One through Four, is cited only when directly quoted and at the beginning of each major section to spare the reader the tedium of a footnote-cluttered page.

The supplemental source most extensively utilized is the oral commentary of the present head of the Ge-luk-ba order, Jam-bel-shen-pen, known as the Gan-den Tri Rin-bo-chay, who is also the former abbot of the Tantric College of Lower Hla-sa (*rgyud med grwa tshang*).[8] As a Visiting Professor and in association with the Center for South Asian Studies of the University of Virginia, Tri Rin-bo-chay taught a series of seminars on the *Illumination of the Texts of Tantra* at the University of Virginia from June, 1980, to July, 1981. Those discourses were recorded and have been partially transcribed. Tri Rin-bo-chay's remarks were profound and extensive, bringing to the text the flavor and insights of the oral tradition. His translator for those seminars was Jeffrey Hopkins, Associate Professor of Northern Buddhism at the University of Virginia and Director of the Center for South Asian Studies, whose incisive questions to Tri Rin-bo-chay resulted often in further clarifications, comparisons, and speculations.

Additional insights and opinions have been gleaned from the writings of several eminent contemporary Ge-luk-ba scholars, including His Holiness Tenzin Gyatso, the Fourteenth Dalai Lama; Geshe Kelsang Gyatso, spiritual director of the Manjushri Institute in England; and Geshe Lhundup Sopa, Professor in the Department of Indian Studies at the University of Wisconsin (Madison). Also, some points have been clarified by reference to Nga-wang-bel-den's chief sources, A-gya Yong-dzin's (*a kya yongs 'dzin*) brief presentation of the grounds and paths of the *Guhyasamāja Tantra*,[9] and the monumental *Great Exposition of Secret*

Mantra by the founder of the Ge-luk-ba order, Dzong-ka-ba
(*tsong kha pa*, 1357–1419).

It has not been my intention to offer original analyses and
reflections on Highest Yoga Tantra, but rather to present
in a simple, straightforward, yet precise fashion, the structure of Highest Yoga Tantra from the point of view of a
single living Buddhist tradition, the Ge-luk-ba school of
Tibet. My focus is entirely on what the Ge-luk-bas think
Highest Yoga Tantra to be about. The reader who wishes to
investigate theories on the origins of tantra or to consider
interpretations of its functions other than those given by the
Ge-luk-ba tradition will need to consult other sources.[10]

Furthermore, the reader should be aware that this presentation of Nga-wang-bel-den's thought on Highest Yoga
Tantra is neither the final word on Highest Yoga Tantra in
Tibet nor even on the Ge-luk-ba school's interpretation of
it. Tibet's other principal Buddhist sects — Nying-ma
(*rnying ma*), Sa-gya (*sa skya*), and Ga-gyu (*bka' brgyud*) —
explain Highest Yoga Tantra somewhat differently, and
even within the Ge-luk-ba tradition there is, on many
points, a diversity of opinions. Nevertheless, the *Illumination of the Texts of Tantra* is a highly regarded text from
within the mainstream of the Ge-luk-ba tradition, the
largest Buddhist school of Tibet, and this partial exegesis of
its contents is offered in the hope that it will serve as a guide
to those interested in Highest Yoga Tantra but put off by
the few dense and difficult studies that now exist, and that
it may yield valuable insights to be applied to future studies
of Buddhist tantra.

It has been decided to present a book based on the
Illumination of the Texts of Tantra rather than a translation at
this time because even though the text is very clear in many
respects, it presupposes extensive background and would
be extremely difficult to read without a lengthy commentary. The present book generally follows the order of topics
in the *Illumination of the Texts of Tantra*, except that a
number of minor points have been eliminated or relegated

to notes in order to prevent the exposition from bogging down; also, Parts One and Two contain much information of an introductory nature that is either not discussed or discussed very briefly by Nga-wang-bel-den.

Despite the obvious importance attached to the practice of tantra by several major Buddhist traditions, Western scholars have written very little on the subject. To date, they have only begun to scratch the surface of an enormous wealth of material extant in Sanskrit and Tibetan. Only a few tantras have been translated, even in part; an even smaller portion of the vast commentarial literature has been examined; and only a few attempts have been made to study Buddhist tantric practice in its contemporary setting.[11]

At the same time, there has clearly been great interest in the subject of tantra. The relative dearth of scholarly studies has been, it seems, largely due to the esoteric nature of the subject. In the first place, tantric texts themselves are open only to those who can read Sanskrit or Tibetan, and, to a lesser extent, Chinese or Japanese, but even the few who have such qualifications are faced with the seemingly insurmountable task of deciphering works encrypted such that they can be understood only by carefully chosen initiates. Moreover, until quite recently, the principal Buddhist practitioners of tantra, the Tibetan Buddhists, severely restricted the dissemination of their accumulated knowledge of tantric practice to outsiders. What little they revealed was carefully prefaced with dire warnings about the extreme danger of revealing the contents of the tantras[12] and was of such a general nature that it could not by itself be used by potential practitioners as a guide to higher practices.

Following the Tibetan diaspora of 1959 onwards, and the resulting dissemination of Tibetan Buddhism to the West, the situation has substantially changed. Recent years have seen the publication of a number of books on tantra in Tibet, some by Tibetans themselves,[13] and a great many Westerners have personally been initiated into tantric practice by Tibetan masters both in India and the West. It seems safe to say that we are now on the threshold of an unprecedented era of explorations of the tantras, and it is hoped that this book will in some small way aid that process by providing a general context for more specialized studies.

Part One
Highest Yoga Tantra
in the Context of Great Vehicle Buddhism

1 The Superiority of Secret Mantra

In general, the vast corpus of Buddhist scriptures may be distinguished into two basic types: sutras and tantras. Traditionally, the sutras are held to be discourses the Buddha spoke openly in his lifetime (c. 560–480 B.C.E.) whereas the tantras are the discourses he, taking the form of various meditational deities or ideal beings,[14] taught secretly to special disciples.[15]

These two divisions of Buddha's word are the scriptural bases for the two "vehicles"* within Great Vehicle Buddhism, the Perfection Vehicle* and the Secret Mantra Vehicle*. The systems based on sutra and tantra are vehicles in the sense that they are the means for traveling to the destinations of either liberation from cyclic existence or to Buddhahood itself.[16] The Perfection Vehicle teaches paths to enlightenment found in the sutra literature, particularly in the Perfection of Wisdom sutras, such as the six perfections* of bodhisattvas. The Secret Mantra Vehicle teaches paths found only in the tantra literature in addition to paths common to sutra and tantra. The Secret Mantra Vehicle's name stems from *mantra**, meaning "mind protection" (*man*, mind + *trā*, protect) in the sense that tantric practice "protects", i.e., isolates, the mind from ordinary appearances through the substitution of exalted appearances.[17]

It is not denied that the presentations of the Buddha's teaching in sutra and tantra sometimes appear to be contradictory, just as his Low Vehicle* and Great Vehicle teachings appear to be contradictory. These putative faults are traditionally cited as indications of the great compassion and singular skill with which the Buddha taught his doctrine according to the widely varying capacities of persons to understand and practice it. It is argued that because a Buddha has at the core of his being the unshakable determination to set all sentient beings in the blissful state of Buddhahood, he teaches everything that might be of help to others, not merely doctrines that can be assimilated by extraordinary individuals. Thus, different systems are developed for different audiences.

The potential hearers of the Buddha's teaching are, in general, said to be of three types: beings of small, middling and great capacity.[18] Beings of small capacity are so-called because they seek only happiness for themselves, either mainly in their present lives or in future lives. Some of those who mainly seek happy future lives are motivated by this goal to practice Buddhism in the most rudimentary fashion by taking refuge in the Three Jewels (the Doctrine, the Teacher — Buddha, and the Spiritual Community*).

Beings of middling capacity have understood the unsatisfactoriness of continued powerless rebirth due to the force of contaminated actions* well enough to have a strong wish to be free from cyclic existence* and suffering. These persons have become capable of entering the practice of the Low Vehicle.

Beings of greatest capacity have not only grasped the benefits of liberation from cyclic existence for themselves, but have been profoundly affected by the realization that what is true for them is true of all others. By reflecting on certain truths, such as that all beings have at one time or another in the vast duration of cyclic existence been their mothers and shown them great kindness, they gradually develop love and compassion for others. Their wish to make others happy and to free them from suffering becomes an "unusual attitude"*, the willingness to take on the burden of bringing all others to the exalted state of Buddhahood. In its highest development, their compassion becomes a determination to achieve Buddhahood as a means for freeing all sentient beings. Beings of greatest capacity are the main trainees of the Great Vehicle, the sutra version of which is also called the Perfection Vehicle*.

Of these altruistic persons, there are some who are very intelligent and at the same time have such great compassion that they cannot bear to spend any unnecessary time in the attainment of Buddhahood because they aspire to be a supreme source of help to others. These persons are said to be qualified to enter the Secret Mantra Vehicle.

According to the Great Vehicle traditions, Buddha set forth several vehicles and innumerable methods and stages so that all beings, whatever their capacity, could progress toward highest enlightenment.[19] That the vehicles and practices differ in completeness or speed is due to the superiority or inferiority of their main trainees. In the Low Vehicle, for instance, the final nature of all phenomena — their absence or emptiness* of inherent existence* — is not taught; only a coarse level of the selflessness of persons is explicitly set forth. The reason, as Chandrakīrti says, is that:[20]

> If emptiness were taught in the very beginning to those who have not developed their intellects, very great ignorance would be produced; therefore, the Superiors* do not teach emptiness in the very beginning.

Similarly, because the main practitioners of the Secret Mantra Vehicle are more intelligent than the main practitioners of the Perfection Vehicle, it is more suitable that they train in the special techniques of tantra.

Both the Perfection Vehicle and the Secret Mantra Vehicle teach practices that are a "union of method and wisdom" (see chart 1). "Wisdom"*, in both vehicles, refers to a consciousness that realizes "emptiness"; emptiness is the lack of inherent existence that every phenomena has as its actual mode of existence.[21] "Method"* refers to motivation and its attendant deeds, which are means of enhancing wisdom. In the Perfection Vehicle the principal method is the practice of the three perfections of giving*, ethics*, and patience*; in the Secret Mantra Vehicle one practices the perfections but also employs "deity yoga"*, causing the mind that directly (non-conceptually) realizes emptiness to appear in the form of a deity such as a Buddha.

Chart 1. *Wisdom and Method*

Vehicle	Wisdom	Method
Perfection Vehicle	Wisdom Consciousness that Realizes Emptiness	Perfections
Secret Mantra Vehicle	Wisdom Consciousness that Realizes Emptiness	Perfections and Deity Yoga

By engaging in the practices of method and wisdom, one builds up the karmic collections of merit* and wisdom that are the causes, respectively, for the two "bodies" of the Buddha, the Form Body* and the Truth Body* (see chart 2). A Buddha's Form Body appears to sentient beings in two ways, as the Complete Enjoyment Body* that always abides in a Highest Pure Land* teaching Bodhisattva Superiors, and as his Emanation Bodies*, a Buddha's appearance spontaneously and instantly throughout the universe in various forms (such as the Buddha Shākyamuni of ancient India) for the sake of all types of sentient beings. Like the Form Body, a Buddha's Truth Body also has two aspects, the Wisdom Body* being the Buddha's omniscient consciousness which remains continually in non-dual meditative equipoise on emptiness, and the Nature Body* being the emptiness — the lack of inherent existence — of that consciousness. The Truth Body is said to be the imprint*, or result, of the collections of wisdom, and the Form Body is said to be the imprint of the collections of merit.

At various times, a Buddha's bodies are enumerated as two, three, four, or more. The two bodies are the Truth Body and the Form Body; the three bodies are the Truth Body, Complete Enjoyment Body, and Emanation Body; and the four bodies are the Wisdom Body, Nature Body, Complete Enjoyment Body, and Emanation Body.

Chart 2. *Bodies of a Buddha*

Truth Body (imprint of wisdom)	Wisdom Body (omniscient consciousness)
	Nature Body (emptiness of Wisdom Body)
Form Body (imprint of merit)	Complete Enjoyment Body
	Emanation Body

It is not possible for either the Form or Truth Bodies of a Buddha to be achieved separately,[22] because attainment of either depends upon the conjoined causal collections of merit and wisdom. Hence, since it is not sufficient to practice only method or only wisdom, all presentations of the path to Buddhahood must explain how method and wisdom are conjoined on the path. On this point, the explanations of the Perfection Vehicle and Secret Mantra Vehicle are significantly different.

When the philosophical tenet systems of the Perfection Vehicle explain the union of method and wisdom on the path, they do not assert that in their systems method and wisdom are an inseparable entity; for them, it is not possible for a single consciousness to realize emptiness explicitly and to engage simultaneously in the practice of giving, and so forth. Rather, they assert that their paths join method and wisdom both in the sense that wisdom — the consciousness that realizes emptiness — is affected by the force of having previously engaged in giving, and so forth, and in the sense that method — the practice of giving, and so forth — is affected by the force of one's having meditated on emptiness.[23]

The texts of the Secret Mantra Vehicle argue that the Perfection Vehicle's conjunction of wisdom and method is merely that of two separate consciousnesses which affect each other, not of a single consciousness in which method and wisdom are mixed. That is why a vast stretch of time — three periods of a countless[24] number of great aeons★ — is required in order to enhance the wisdom consciousness that realizes emptiness so that it is able to overcome all forms of the extremely tenacious and pervasive conception of inherent existence and the predispositions it establishes, which together comprise the two types of obstructions barring the way to full enlightenment. In fact, according to Highest Yoga Tantra, even three periods of a countless number of great aeons spent in the practice of the Perfection Vehicle are insufficient for the attainment of Buddhahood; without engaging in tantric practice, one is destined to ascend no higher than the tenth Bodhisattva ground, the last gradation of the path prior to Buddhahood.[25]

The Secret Mantra Vehicle teaches deity yoga, an extraordinary method of uniting wisdom and method in which wisdom and method are joined together in a single consciousness. The subtle consciousness used to realize emptiness appears in compassionate physical form (a Form Body), thus uniting wisdom and compassionate method in a single consciousness, called deity yoga. Through this, one is able to amass simultaneously the requisite collections of merit and wisdom, making it possible to attain Buddhahood in less than three periods of countless aeons.[26] In Highest Yoga Tantra, Buddhahood can be attained in as little as one lifetime. Deity yoga is the principal method that the tantras add to Perfection Vehicle practices; hence, all of the specific

techniques taught in the tantras are said by Dzong-ka-ba to
be "either methods for heightening cognition of emptiness
or branches of deity yoga."[27]
Deity yoga surpasses the practice of the perfections of
giving, and so forth, by being a union of wisdom and
method in one consciousness, but it also is superior to the
methods of the Perfection Vehicle because it is a technique
that actually *resembles* the countenance, or aspect*, of the
Form Body of a Buddha. In other words, giving, patience,
and ethics are admitted to be powerful practices, but because they bear no resemblance to a Buddha's marvelous
Form Body, they cannot develop into it. The unique
method of Secret Mantra, on the other hand, is to cause
one's own mind, absorbed in the realization of emptiness,
to appear in the form of the very enlightened being — a
Buddha — that one is destined to become upon
enlightenment.[28] This compassionate appearance of the
mind that realizes emptiness, in the form of a Buddha deity,
actually develops into the Form Body of a Buddha while the
mind itself develops into the Truth Body of a Buddha. As
the current Dalai Lama succinctly says, "In brief, the Body
of a Buddha is attained through meditating on it."[29]
Highest Yoga Tantra comprises two stages, the stage of
generation* and the stage of completion. Both are concerned with the transformation of one's mind and body
into the mind and body of a Buddha. On the stage of generation, one generates a vivid imaginative visualization of one's
transformation into a deity; then, the stage of completion
"completes" the transformation by actually bringing about
a new physical structure, that is, by transforming one into
an actual deity, a Buddha. Deity yoga, in general, is such a
powerful transformative technique that even the stage of
generation, in which one merely visualizes a deity, is said to
far surpass the Perfection Vehicle in terms of its capacity to
overcome the obstructions to enlightenment. Kay-drup
(*mkhas grub*), one of the two chief disciples of Dzong-ka-ba,
the founder of the Ge-luk-ba order, explains the great dif-

ference it makes to meditate on emptiness using a divine image rather than an ordinary object:[30]

> In terms of capacity to serve as an antidote to the consciousness conceiving inherent existence, that mind which, observing a divine circle [of deities and their divine environment], ascertains the object of observation — the absence of inherent existence — surpasses one hundred-fold an awareness such as that which, observing a sprout, ascertains the absence of inherent existence.

The mind accomplished by deity yoga — one which realizes emptiness at the same time it compassionately appears as a deity — is not even considered possible in the Perfection Vehicle, where it is usually said that when emptiness is realized, the subject whose emptiness is being realized does not itself appear to the mind.[31] However, according to Ge-luk-ba scholars, it is possible for two factors — the factor of ascertainment, which realizes emptiness, and the factor of appearance, which appears as a divine body — to exist simultaneously within the entity of one consciousness; in other words, they claim that the mind that realizes emptiness itself can appear in the form of a deity.

2 Paths Common to Sutra and Tantra

As mentioned earlier, Highest Yoga Tantra practice comprises two stages, the stage of generation and the stage of completion. The stage of completion is necessarily preceeded by the stage of generation, which itself has three sets of prerequisites: (1) previous practice of the paths common to sutra and tantra; (2) initiation★ in a tantra of the Highest Yoga Tantra set; and (3) assuming special tantric pledges★ and vows★. Before beginning to describe the stage of generation in detail, these three sets of prerequisites will be briefly explained.

Before practicing the stages of Highest Yoga Tantra, it is necessary to establish in one's mind the correct motivation and the correct view as taught in the sutra presentations of the paths to enlightenment. Indeed, almost all of the features of sutra are included in tantra;[32] hence, the tantras do not replace the sutras, but rather, complement them. That being the case, the three principal aspects of the path, as delineated by the Indian scholar Atisha and explained by Dzong-ka-ba and many others, are no less indispensible to tantric practitioners than they are to others. The three principal aspects of the path are: (1) *renunciation*★, the determination to leave cyclic existence; (2) *the altruistic aspira-*

*tion to enlightenment**, the determination to become a Buddha for the sake of all sentient beings; and (3) *the correct view**, the realization that all phenomena are empty of inherent existence.

The Need for Renunciation

Those who aspire to enlightenment must turn away from their attachment to the appearances of this life and their attachment to future lives, meditating on the meaningfulness of leisure and fortune and the difficulty of finding it and the inevitability of suffering and death. It is said that without a strong intention to renounce cyclic existence there is no way to generate a strong aspiration to attain Buddhahood. As Dzong-ka-ba says in his *Three Principal Aspects of the Path* (*lam gyi gtso bo rnam pa gsum*):[33]

> Without a complete thought definitely to leave
> Cyclic existence there is no way to stop
> Seeking pleasurable effects in the ocean of
>   existence.
> Also, craving cyclic existence thoroughly binds
> The embodied; therefore, in the beginning, a
>   thought
> Definitely to leave cyclic existence should be
>   sought.

Renunciation is a prerequisite for the practice of any vehicle, be it sutra or tantra. For tantra, renunciation is particularly important because sexual desire is used in the path; without renunciation, the practitioner can easily become attached to the object of desire.[34]

The Need for Compassion

Tantric trainees, like Perfection Vehicle trainees, should be Bodhisattvas**, persons who not only have renounced the world, but are fully committed to attaining enlightenment in order to serve the welfare of others.[35] In fact, those who practice tantra should have an extraordinary degree of com-

passion; their motivation for practicing tantra should be
that they cannot bear to spend unnecessary time attaining
Buddhahood because they want to be a supreme source of
help and happiness to others as soon as possible.[36] As
Jang-gya (*lcang skya*, 1717-86) says in his *Presentation of
Tenets (grub mtha'i rnam bzhag)*:[37]

> It is said in the precious tantras and in many com-
> mentaries that even those trainees of the Mantra
> Vehicle who have low faculties must have far great-
> er compassion, sharper faculties, and a superior lot
> than the trainees of sharpest faculties in the Perfec-
> tion Vehicle.

Jang-gya contradicts a view, widely held in the West,[38] that
compassion belongs to an earlier phase of Buddhism, tantra
having replaced compassion with passion.

The Need for Wisdom
Tantric practitioners should also have made progress in
meditation on emptiness. Meditation on emptiness is the
heart of the Buddhist path in both sutra and tantra.
Although compassion is said to be the basis of practice, it is
basic in the sense of being one's motivation; meditation on
emptiness is the chief practice of Buddhism because it
actualizes one's compassionate intent by removing all obstructions to Buddhahood. All the practices of method,
both in sutra and tantra, are done specifically in order to
enhance the wisdom consciousness that realizes emptiness,
as Shāntideva's *Engaging in the Bodhisattva Deeds (spyod
'jug, bodhicaryavatara*, IX.1) says:[39]

> The Subduer said that all these
> Branches are for the sake of wisdom.

Considering the centrality of meditation on emptiness to the
tantric path, it must be regarded as misleading to contrast
the Secret Mantra Vehicle to the Perfection Vehicle as does
S.B. Dasgupta:[40]

The different metaphysical systems deal with the nature of reality and the philosophical method for its realization; whereas the tantras lay stress on the esoteric methods for realizing that reality.

On the contrary, Jeffrey Hopkins argues the tantric yogi must engage in the same sort of reasonings as other Buddhist practitioners:[41]

> ... non-dualistic wisdom is the life of both the sutra and tantra paths, and in both paths initial reliance on reasoning to uncover the nature of phenomena, hidden to our direct experience, is necessary.

Tantric yogis succeed in their cultivation of wisdom more quickly than do practitioners of the Perfection Vehicle because the tantric yogi, employing deity yoga, can achieve a mind that is a union of calm abiding★ and special insight★ — a mind of alert one-pointedness that realizes emptiness — in far less time than the period of countless great aeons required for those who practice sutra paths alone.[42] Tantric yogis use deity yoga to enhance meditation on emptiness; their use of deity yoga brings them more quickly to an initial direct cognition of emptiness by enhancing their ability to combine meditative stability with analysis (see pp. 55–6). Also, in Highest Yoga Tantra, powerful, subtle consciousnesses that realize emptiness are manifested, whereby the obstructions to liberation★ and omniscience★ are quickly overcome.

Even though tantric practitioners seem to be superior to others both in terms of their cultivation of method and their cultivation of wisdom, some commentators, both past and present, have thought that they are inferior. For instance, the great Italian Tibetologist, Guiseppe Tucci, says:[43]

> The tantras of the 'superior class' are above all addressed to men in whom non-religious impulses, especially those of a sexual nature, are at their most powerful.

Also:[44]

> The *Anuttaratantras* are reserved for the creatures who sin most, who do not distinguish good from evil, who lead impure lives.

Notions such as these are explicitly refuted by Ge-luk-ba scholars. Practitioners of tantra, they say, should be acting on the purest of motives — the altruistic aspiration to highest enlightenment — and should have impeccable behavior. Highest Yoga Tantra does indeed use desire, but only to destroy desire, just as "wood-born" insects eat the wood that engenders them.[45] Desire is used to generate a powerful bliss consciousness which is then employed in the destruction of the root of desire, the conception of inherent existence, through realizing the emptiness of inherent existence.

Ge-luk-ba scholars also reject the position that tantra is an easy path, meant for persons incapable of more difficult practices, as Mircea Eliade has suggested:[46] "... the Vajrayāna represents a new revelation of Buddha's doctrine adapted to the much diminished capacities of modern man." On the contrary, the tantric path is considered far more difficult than the sutra path. Consequently, it is said that there are many who wish to practice tantra but few who are qualified for it.[47]

3 Initiation

In addition to cultivating renunciation, compassion, and the correct view, the practice of the stage of generation of a particular tantra requires that one must first receive an initiation*[48] from a fully-qualified master of that tantra. An initiation is a rite involving extensive visualization, prayers, offerings, and the use of ritual implements and substances, its purpose being to purify defilements, to confer upon initiates permission to practice the tantra, to teach them the procedure of the stages of practice, and to establish in them potencies for successful practice.

To practice the path fully, one needs four types of initiations: the vase initiation*, the secret initiation*, the knowledge-wisdom initiation*, and the word initiation* (see chart 3, p. 36). The vase initiation, which is conferred by means of water from a vase, is given in all four tantra sets, whereas the latter three initiations are unique to Highest Yoga Tantra.[49] Only the vase initiation is necessary in order to practice the stage of generation; the remaining three initiations are bestowed prior to embarking on the stage of completion.

The vase initiation is a rite involving one of four types of mandalas*:[50] a painted cloth mandala, a colored sand mandala, a body mandala, or a concentration mandala. A mandala is a "divine circle"; the term can refer either to a specific deity or to the deity's habitat. "Mandala" is also frequently used to designate a representation in two or three dimensions of the inestimable mansion and surroundings of a particular deity. A painted cloth mandala is a two-dimensional painted rendering of the deity's marvelous mansion and its inhabitants, usually hung on a wall, and a colored sand mandala is a similar representation drawn on a platform or floor with colored sand particles tapped from sand muskets. Body mandalas, in which the lama's body is visualized as the parts of the mandala,[51] are less frequently used due to certain restrictions: (1) they cannot be used with one who has not initially received initiation in the tantra by some other means; (2) though they are acknowledged in the *Guhyasamāja Tantra*, they are not used for initiation; and (3) they do not exist at all in the three lower tantras and some Highest Yoga Tantras such as *Vajrabhairava* (*rdo rje 'jigs byed*). Concentration mandalas — visualized mandalas that appear clearly both to a lama and his student as a result of their individual concentrations — are even rarer.[52]

The secret, knowledge-wisdom, and word initiations, when given in their full-fledged form using actual substances and consorts, are given only to special highly advanced trainees.[53] The secret initiation involves the use of a "conventional mind of enlightenment"* mandala, the conventional mind of enlightenment being a mixture of the fluids of the male and female deities produced by sexual union. Similarly, the wisdom initiation involves the use of a "vagina"* mandala.[54] The word initiation involves the use of an "ultimate mind of enlightenment"* mandala, this being the words of instruction given by the lama concerning the union of pure body and pure mind.[55]

There are four levels of attainment of initiation.[56] The lowest level of attainment of initiation is to pretend that when the initiation is bestowed, bliss is generated. The

Chart 3. *Initiations*

Type of Initiation	Mandala	Practice that is Authorized
Vase Initiation	Painted Cloth, Sand, Body or Concentration Mandala	Highest Yoga Tantra in General
Secret Initiation	Conventional Mind of Enlightenment Mandala	Illusory Body
Wisdom Initiation	Vagina Mandala	Clear Light
Word Initiation	Ultimate Mind of Enlightenment Mandala	Union

second is to develop some bliss from the touch of the water or other initiation implement at the time of initiation. The third is to mimic meditation on emptiness with a consciousness of great bliss. The greatest is actually to experience great bliss from the bestowal of initiation and to use that bliss consciousness to meditate on emptiness.

4 Pledges and Vows[57]

At the time of initiation, tantric practitioners take various vows and make pledges in addition to those they share with Perfection Vehicle trainees. Among these promises are a pledge of secrecy, for tantric practices are not only difficult, but dangerous (because engaging in practices involving desire without having established a pure motivation would only increase one's afflictive karma).

All tantric practitioners must take and protect the eighteen root and forty-six auxilliary Bodhisattva vows. Additionally, in Yoga Tantra and in Highest Yoga Tantra, there are fourteen root and ten additional tantric vows. Thus, it is hardly the case, as some have thought,[58] that tantric yogis are lawless. Their behavior is, in fact, strictly regulated.

For each tantra in the Highest Yoga Tantra class, there are specific pledges — promises to engage in various practices of ethical behavior — and vows — promises *not* to engage in certain forms of behavior — to be taken at the time of receiving initiation. In the *Kālachakra Tantra*, for instance, there are twenty-five modes of behavior that are to be guarded against: five ill-deeds (taking life, taking what is not given, adultery, lying, and drinking beer), five secondary ill-deeds (making bets, playing dice, eating impure flesh, senseless chatter, dispersing offerings to ancestors, and cow-sacrifice), five killings (of ox, child, woman, man, or [Buddha-] images), five wrong thoughts (non-faith in the Buddha and his Doctrine, malice towards leaders, malice towards the Spiritual Community, and cheating those who trust one), and five desires (for forms, sounds, odors, tastes, and tangible objects).[59]

These pledges and vows differ slightly from tantra to tantra, but in every case, keeping the pledges and vows is held to be extremely important. It is said that even if one does not practice the tantric paths with great effort, but manages to keep the pledges and vows, one will attain Buddhahood in no more than sixteen lifetimes.[60] On the other hand, if one does not keep the pledges and vows, no matter how well one performs the other practices, one will fall into a bad migration.[61]

If the pledges or vows are broken, they may be reinstated by following a ritual procedure specified in the tantra for disclosing the infractions and by promising to refrain from future repetition of them.

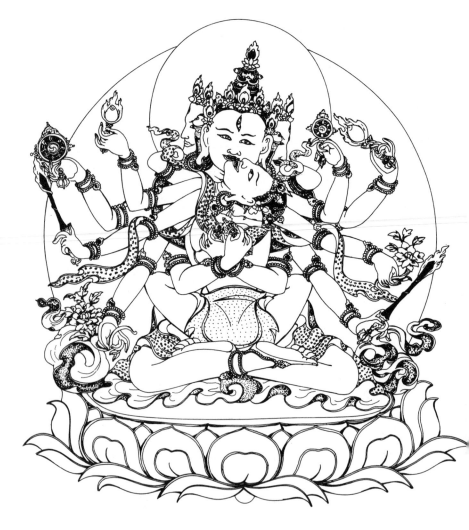

Guhyasamāja

1 Features of the Stage of Generation

The purpose of the stage of generation is to "ripen" the mental continuum* for the stage of completion. Its synonyms include "stage of imagination"* and "yoga of fabrication"*.[62] It is a rehearsal of the stage of completion in the sense that one passes from the stage of generation to the stage of completion by bringing one's imaginative vision to such a height of clarity and power that what one has imagined begins to become real. The stage of completion "completes" the vision by effecting the transformation of the trainee into a Buddha.

The definition of the stage of generation is:[63]

> A yoga that (1) does *not* arise from causing the winds to enter, abide, and dissolve in the central channel through the power of meditation but is a ripener of the continuum for the stage of completion that is its effect and (2) is a meditation newly and mentally imagining an aspect similar to any of the three — birth, death, and intermediate state.

The remainder of this section will explain the key terms of this definition.

Yogas

"Yoga"★ is derived from the Sanskrit root *yuj*, to join; it is cognate with the English word "yoke".[64] In general, yoga means to control the mind, to join one's mind to a fact.[65] In the context of Highest Yoga Tantra, yoga also refers to the union, in one consciousness, of the sublime and the profound — a sublime feeling of bliss combined with the profound realization that persons and other phenomena lack inherent existence.[66] The generation of this consciousness, in which the feeling of bliss is mixed with emptiness such that they seem to be undifferentiable, is the greatest achievement of tantric practice. With a powerful, subtle composite of bliss and the realization of emptiness it is possible to overcome the obstructions barring the way to Buddhahood in as little as one lifetime, whereas no non-tantric practice enables the accomplishment of this goal in less than three periods of countless great aeons.

Yogas of the stages of Highest Yoga Tantra induce path consciousnesses — minds comprising the five paths of accumulation★, preparation★, seeing★, meditation★, and no more learning★, the stages of progression towards Buddhahood (see chart 4, p. 62). Practitioners on the first four paths are called "learners", for they strive towards but have not yet reached the level of Buddhahood, the "path of no more learning".

Winds

The yogas of the two stages of Highest Yoga Tantra are performed in order to control "winds"★, or vital energies. In Buddhist physiology, the winds are not merely moving air, but are the vital energies that cause all movement by and within the body, such as muscular movement, the circulation of blood and lymph, defecation and urination, breathing, and so forth.

The winds also are instrumental in the functioning of the six consciousnesses or minds (ear, eye, nose, tongue, body, and mental).[67] Consciousnesses are said to "ride" on winds in the same manner that a horseman rides his mount; by travelling on the winds, consciousnesses are able to leave their bases in the sense-powers (located in the eye, ear, and so forth) to contact their objects. Because minds are inoperative without winds to provide a medium for their movement, and because winds lack specific direction without minds, minds are likened to cripples with sight and winds to blind men with legs;[68] the lame climb on the backs of the blind and together they can move about. Because the winds are the medium for the operation of minds, fluctuation in the winds necessarily affects consciousness, and thus it is crucial for tantric yogis who wish to yoke consciousness to gain control over the movement of winds. Tantric yogis engage in a variety of practices to bring about a concentration of the winds, for concentration of the winds leads to concentration of consciousness.

The winds are distinguished in several different ways in Nga-wang-bel-den's description of the stages of Highest Yoga Tantra. In one scheme, winds are enumerated as five: (1) the vitalizing wind*, which causes inhalation, exhalation, and so forth; (2) the pervasive wind*, which makes possible the movement of the limbs, and so forth; (3) the upward-moving wind*, which is involved in speech, swallowing, and so forth; (4) the downward-voiding wind*, which is responsible for defecation, urination, the emission of semen, and so forth; and (5) the fire-dwelling wind*, which is responsible for digestion, and so forth.[69]

In another scheme, winds are distinguished into basic winds* and secondary winds*; the basic winds are the five winds just mentioned, and the secondary winds are the five parts of the vitalizing wind which are associated with the five senses.[70] (Thus, the secondary winds are actually included within the basic winds.)

In yet another scheme, winds are divided into coarse winds and subtle winds. Of those two, only the coarse winds (the coarse basic and secondary winds) operate in ordinary waking life.[71] The subtle winds are the basis for mind of clear light*, and hence for the illusory body* (both of which will be explained later), and operate only after all the coarse winds have dissolved.

Channels

The winds move in a system of 72,000 subtle "channels"* arrayed throughout the body.[72] There are three major channels, running parallel to each other from mid-forehead up over the crown of the head down to the base of the spine and then under the trunk of the body to the tip of the sexual organ. The upper opening of the central channel* is at the forehead between the eyes and the upper openings of the right channel* and left channel* are at the top of the nose.[73]

The right channel and left channel wrap around the central channel at certain places, constricting it such that the winds cannot pass through it. In the *Guhyasamāja* system, the central channel is said to have seven loci of constriction; they are called channel-wheels* because many smaller channels branch out of them like the spokes of a wheel, and they are also called channel-knots* because of being places of constriction.[74] The wheel-spokes are sometimes called petals because the channel-wheel spreads out like a flower.

The channel-wheels are located at the forehead, the crown of the head, the throat, the heart, the navel, the "secret place", and the opening or tip of the sexual organ.[75] The forehead channel-wheel is the upper opening of the central channel and the channel-wheel at the tip of the sexual organ is its lower opening. The navel channel-wheel is located behind the solar plexus, closer to the spine than the navel. The "secret place" is located at the base of the spine. The channel-wheels have varying numbers of petals or spokes: at the crown there are thirty-two petals, at the throat there are sixteen, at the heart there are eight, at the navel there are sixty-four, at the "secret place" there are thirty-two, and at the sexual organ there are eight.[76]

Winds can move both into and out of the central channel

at any of the channel wheels, not merely at just the upper and lower openings. However, the same knots that constrict the vertical movement of winds in the central channel also "plug" the central channel ends of the spokes or petals. Until the knots at the channel wheels are loosened, winds from various parts of the body may be drawn up to those places but not past them; for instance, at the end of the practice of physical isolation, the winds are drawn into the central channel but cannot enter the heart because of the heart channel-knot.[77]

The sign that winds have entered the central channel is that the pressure of exhalation and inhalation is equal and that the volume and pressure of air moving in each nostril is equal, whereas normally there are various imbalances in the breath.[78] As more winds enter the central channel, breathing becomes progressively weaker and finally ceases altogether.

Dissolution of Winds
In the context of the three lower tantra sets — Action Tantra, Performance Tantra, and Yoga Tantra — gaining control over the winds means to be able to restrain the senses by preventing the winds they depend on from going out of the "doors" (the eyes, ears, and so forth) of the senses. However, in Highest Yoga Tantra, the aim is not merely to prevent the winds from going outside, but actually to draw them into the body and then into the central channel by the power of meditation. When the winds are caused to enter the central channel, they are held there, moved around, and drawn into various places where they "dissolve" (cease). The dissolution or cessation of winds concomitantly causes the cessation of the types of minds that rely upon them. Thus, as the coarser winds cease, so do the coarser types of minds, leaving only subtle winds and minds.[79] The remaining subtle mind (mounted on the remaining subtle wind) is then used to cognize emptiness.

The Power of Meditation

The meditation that causes the winds to enter, remain, and dissolve in the central channel consists of special techniques involving penetrative focusing on important parts of the body. The practice of penetrative focusing is begun on the stage of generation, but at that time it is not yet developed sufficiently to cause the entry and dissolution of winds in the central channel. That is what occurs on the stage of completion.

In addition to the techniques involving intensive focusing, yogis of the stage of completion use sexual union with either a real or imagined consort to generate sexual desire, which in turn is used to enhance concentration and cause the generation of a blissful physical and mental feeling. The bliss thus engendered causes the manifestation of subtle consciousnesses called "empties" which the yogis use to realize emptiness. Then, after meditation on emptiness, they practice perceiving all phenomena to be manifestations of bliss and emptiness.

Through lengthy cultivation of these practices over the various levels of the two stages of Highest Yoga Tantra, one completes the collections of merit and wisdom, the imprints of which are the Form and Truth Bodies of a Buddha. These techniques will be described in subsequent chapters on the levels of the stage of completion.

Death, Intermediate State, and Rebirth

By gaining control over the winds, yogis mimic the process of death, intermediate state*, and rebirth.[80] They are then able to actualize subtle consciousnesses capable of overcoming the barriers to full enlightenment.

In the process of ordinary death, winds are involuntarily drawn into the central channel, the channel knots relax, and those winds dissolve into the indestructible drop in the center of the heart. This causes the manifestation of the most subtle of all consciousnesses, the mind of clear light.[81] When the mind of clear light of death ceases, the intermediate state commences, and rebirth occurs some-time within the following forty-nine days.[82]

Special meditative techniques are used in both stages of Highest Yoga Tantra to bring about the same sequence of events as in ordinary death. During the stage of completion, winds enter the central channel, remain there, and then dissolve into the indestructible drop; concurrently, the mind of clear light dawns. However, because these events occur due to the power of meditation one does not enter the intermediate state as one would subsequent to death; rather, one rises in an illusory body — an unobstructive, subtle body made of wind that resembles a deity — and instead of being powerlessly reborn into cyclic existence*, one eventually becomes a Buddha.

Most of the meditations of the stage of generation mimic the process of death, intermediate state, and rebirth, as specified in the definition, but, according to Nga-wang-bel-den, some do not. For instance, yogas of the stage of generation are said to include the use of an actual consort or the visualization of a circle of protective deities, but neither of those are practices that mimic death, intermediate state, and rebirth.[83]

2 Divisions of the Stage of Generation

There are numerous ways to divide the stage of generation. As in the three lower tantra sets — Action Tantra, Performance Tantra, and Yoga Tantra — one can speak in Highest Yoga Tantra of "four branches of approximation and achievement," or "four yogas," or "six branches," or "three meditative stabilizations".[84] The *Illumination of the Texts of Tantra* describes fully only two of these ways to distinguish the phases of the stage of generation, a division into coarse and subtle stages of generation and a division into three meditative stabilizations. However, it also sets forth a division of the persons on the path in terms of their mastery of practice, particularly visualization practice, that illuminates aspects of practice on the stage of generation. Those three modes of division will be described in this section.

Coarse and Subtle Yogas

The "coarse" stage of generation is the "yoga of single-mindedness of the coarse,"*[85] a practice involving the visualization of imaginary deities and their divine residence, which together are called the coarse mandala. The mandala is considered "coarse" not because it lacks clarity or detail, but simply to distinguish it from the mandala imagined on the subtle stage of generation. On the subtle stage of generation, an entire mandala full of deities and other features is visualized inside a tiny drop.

The visualization of the coarse mandala is called a yoga of single-mindedness to indicate that one is to focus intensively on the mandala, building up a mental image of the various deities, architectural and ornamental features, and larger environment. Dzong-ka-ba says:[86]

> The phrase "single-mindedness" refers neither to one occasion of being mindful of the deity, nor to mindfulness of just one deity. Rather, it is mindfulness of only the deity, or mindfulness of oneself and the deity as one. Though in general that [term] applies to meditating on both coarse and subtle deities, here it is the coarse yoga of divine residence and residents... When one trains in the stage of generation, one initially generates a meditative stabilization in which the coarse appears clearly.

The visualization proceeds in accordance with a specific tantra's "means of achievement,"* its *sādhana*; this is a meditation manual written to facilitate visualization. The vision of the mandala is to be built up in each meditative session by adding on pieces until the whole is achieved; one does the entire "means of achievement" in each meditative session, not just a portion.

For example, if one were practicing the stage of generation of the *Kālachakra Tantra*,[87] one would need to imagine oneself as Kālachakra, as follows. One's body is dark blue, with three necks of black, red, and white, and four faces of black, red, white, and yellow, each with three eyes. One's hair is bound on the top of one's head, and one's crown is ornamented with a vajra, a half moon, and a figure of Vajrasattva. Various ornaments — earrings, garlands, and so forth — adorn one's body. There are twelve upper arms — two red arms, two blue arms, and two white arms on each side — and twenty-four lower arms — four black arms, four red arms, and four white arms on each side. One's hands respectively hold a vajra, a sword, a trident, a curved knife, a triple arrow, a vajra hook, a drum, a mallet, a wheel, a spear, a staff, an axe, a bell, a shield, a khaṭvāṅga (a three-pointed instrument), a skull filled with blood, a bow, a noose, a jewel, a lotus, a conch, a mirror, an iron chain, and a four-faced head of Brahmā. One leg is red, the other white; one's right foot treads on a Cupid, the other on a Rudra. Kālachakra embraces his consort Vishvamātā, whose body is yellow, with four faces of yellow, white, blue, and red, each with three eyes. She has four arms on each side, which respectively hold a curved knife, an iron hook, a drum, a rosary, a skull, a noose, a white lotus, and a jewel.

Additionally, since Kālachakra and Vishvamātā are three deities in one, one would imagine Akshobhya and Vajrasattva, who are fused with Kālachakra, and Vajradhatvîshvarî and Prajñāramitā, who are fused with Vishvamātā, as they would look when separated from Kālachakra and Vishvamātā. One would also imagine the ten goddesses — *shaktis* — who stand on the petals of a lotus beneath the central deities. Accomplishing the visualization of all this, one would still only have begun to visualize the multitude of deities, a total of seven hundred twenty-two, that abide in the various parts of the mandala. Also, the mandala itself, in which the deities appear, is an extremely elaborate building with five tiers and extensive grounds. For instance, each of the four walls of this building has an elaborate doorway in the alcoves of which are many objects and beings.

Such is a brief indication of the visualization performed on the coarse stage of generation. In the subtle stage of generation, the "yoga conceiving the subtle,"* one imagines that the entire mandala is contained within a tiny drop, the drop being located at the upper or lower opening of the central channel. With the perfection of this yoga through the attainment of calm abiding and special insight (see pp.

55–6), one moves from the stage of generation to the stage of completion.

Three Meditative Stabilizations

Another way to distinguish phases of the stage of generation is by way of the three meditative stabilizations. The three meditative stabilizations are a way of describing the various degrees of accomplishment in visualization. The first of these three is "initial application"*, in which one works on generating the clear appearance of the divine environment and the basic figures of the mandala; the second is "supreme king of mandalas,"* in which one generates the full mandala; and the third is "supreme king of actions,"*[88] in which one imaginatively acts as the deity, doing various activities such as purifying places and beings.

Throughout all three meditative stabilizations, one is to maintain cognition of emptiness. Dzong-ka-ba says:[89]

> The yoga in which the mind possessing the aspect of a [divine] circle is absorbed in suchness, that is to say, selflessness, is, in accordance with Bel-dray-dor-jay's (*dpal 'bras rdo rje*) explanation, the general procedure of all three meditative stabilizations. Such is also the thought of Jñānapāda. At the time of the first stage [i.e., the initial visualization of deities], meditation on the circle of deities — the class of the appearing — is indeed main. However, through inducing strong force of ascertainment with respect to the meaning of the non-inherent existence of phenomena, one trains in [causing] everything to appear as like illusions. And after meditating on the divine circle, one is to do — with each cultivation of clear realization — the yoga of non-dual profundity and manifestation in which the mind having observed the object of observation, the deity, has the [subjective] aspect of ascertaining the meaning of the absence of inherent existence. The

mode of apprehension of the ascertaining consciousness is absorbed in suchness and that which has the
aspect of the apprehended [i.e., that consciousness]
appears in the aspect of the deities of the support
and supported.

The visualization of deities on the stage of generation, no
matter which of the three meditative stabilizations one is
practicing, must include cognition of emptiness. As Dzong-
ka-ba says, the mind observing a deity is at one and the
same time absorbed in the realization of emptiness and is
itself appearing as the deity under observation.

Four Levels of Achievement

Persons traversing the two stages of Highest Yoga Tantra
are often designated according to the level of the path they
have achieved, but they are also sometimes designated
according to a broader four-fold scheme: (1) beginners*, (2)
those on whom a little wisdom has descended*, (3) those
who have attained slight mastery with respect to wisdom*,
and (4) those who have attained thorough mastery with
respect to wisdom*.[90] In terms of the stages of generation
and completion, beginners and those upon whom a little
wisdom has descended are practitioners of the coarse stage
of generation; those who have attained a slight mastery with
respect to wisdom range from practitioners of the subtle
stage of generation through to practitioners at the end of the
level of impure illusory body in the stage of completion; and
those who have attained thorough mastery with respect to
wisdom are practitioners who have attained at least the level
of clear light of the stage of completion.

Beginners are yogis who have not yet managed to make
the entire coarse mandala appear clearly for at least forty-
eight minutes.[91] Given the tremendous detail in a typical
mandala (for instance, *Guhyasamāja* has thirty-two major
deities, each with smaller deity figures located at their sense
organs, in addition to the many other features of the divine

mansion and its grounds) one is likely to remain a "beginner" for a long time, though a year is said to be sufficient if one works at it continuously.[92] A beginner works serially, building up the various parts of the image one at a time while performing the entire visualization in every session.

Those upon whom a little wisdom has descended are able to visualize clearly and firmly the entire coarse mandala with all its deities — with arms, legs, and most minor features — at one time. However, they are as yet unable to cause the tiny deities located at the sense organs of the major deities to appear clearly. They can cause the entire *coarse* mandala to appear suddenly, but they are still working by stages on the addition of the subtle deities. Wisdom "descends" in the sense that at this level one imagines that visualized deities enter one's ordinary body through the top of the head and dissolve there, causing a special feeling, like goose bumps.[93]

Those who have attained slight mastery with respect to wisdom are able to visualize clearly and firmly the entire mandala, even the subtle deities at the sense organs of the larger deities, at one time. They have by this stage become so familiar with the images visualized that those images can appear with the slightest effort; thus, it is said that it is no longer necessary to distinguish meditative sessions from non-sessions, since one can do deity yoga at all times, maintaining the sense that one is a deity while carrying out all manner of daily activities. At higher levels, even one's need for ordinary nourishment diminishes; one "lives off the food of meditative stabilization."[94] Those who have attained slight mastery with respect to wisdom have reached at least the subtle stage of generation, where the emphasis changes from simply visualizing the mandala in normal size to shrinking it so that the entire mandala appears in a tiny drop or hand-held symbol (such as a vajra or lotus).[95]

Finally, those who have attained thorough mastery with respect to wisdom have attained at least the actual clear light of the stage of completion.[96] At that point, their cultivation

3 Calm Abiding and Special Insight

In the course of the visualization practices of the coarse and subtle stages of generation, it is necessary to analyze again and again.[97] That is, one must establish and re-establish the parts of the visualized mandala of deities and inestimable mansion by recalling from memory their color, placements, names, and so forth, and one must think again and again that they are divine appearances. Also, one must adjust and balance the appearance of the image.[98]

In general, analysis tends to destroy the stability of one's concentration on an object, just as stability tends to preclude analysis. In the system of the Perfection Vehicle, it is not until well after one has attained calm abiding* — a state of strong, pliant meditative stabilization* in which it is possible to remain for as long as one wishes on a certain object of observation — that analysis no longer impedes stability but actually works to promote it. In that system, after one attains calm abiding, one alternates meditation on emptiness and the cultivation of meditative stabilization until familiarity with both makes it possible to perform strong analysis without destroying stability. It is said that eventually, analysis will even induce greater stability.

In tantra, however, even during the stage of generation

analysis can promote, rather than destroy, stability, making it possible to attain calm abiding without refraining from analysis and to attain a union of calm abiding and special insight* very quickly.[99] Special insight is a conceptual or direct realization of emptiness occurring within a state arisen from meditation, i.e., a conceptual or direct realization of emptiness by a mind with the stability of at least the level of calm abiding.

In the context of tantra, a union of calm abiding and special insight is gained through the practice of withdrawal and dispersal of visualized deities.[100] This practice is performed within meditation on emptiness in the sense that it is imagined that the deities are one's own wisdom consciousness that realizes emptiness and simultaneously appears in those forms. However, one is not analyzing an object's mode of existence, as one does in the Perfection Vehicle.[101] There is, therefore, no alternation of practices leading to stability and those leading to wisdom such as in the Perfection Vehicle; both are carried out at the same time with the same consciousness.

This meditative stabilization is brought about by two practices. (1) Initially, one meditates on a subtle drop, visualized as containing an entire mandala of deities, located at the upper opening of the central channel (the location of the forehead channel-wheel). When that meditation becomes stable, calm abiding is attained.[102] (2) One then visualizes that deities are emanated from the subtle drop out into the world in a number equal to the number of sentient beings in order to be of help to those beings, and then visualizes the withdrawal of those deities back into the drop.[103] By the repeated practice of the dispersal and withdrawal of deities, a union of calm abiding and special insight is achieved, and the stage of generation is brought to conclusion.

4 Divine Pride

To this point, the description of the stage of generation has emphasized one's appearance as a deity, but of at least as much importance is the cultivation of what is called "divine pride". As was mentioned earlier, the very meaning of "mantra" in "Secret Mantra" is protection of the mind from ordinary appearance and from conceiving oneself to be ordinary. In the systems of Secret Mantra, one protects the mind from ordinariness by combining visualization of purity — the divine mansion and its divine inhabitants — with "divine pride", the thought that one is oneself the deity being visualized.[104] In fact, the development of divine pride is said to be the main practice of the stage of generation, the cultivation of divine appearances being of secondary importance. The two are, of course, closely connected and mutually supportive.

The cultivation of divine pride is begun right at the inception of the coarse stage of generation, for "single-mindedness" with respect to the coarse mandala of deities and their mansion means to adhere firmly to the notion that one is the deity being visualized. As one gains facility in visualization, the mind becomes entirely absorbed in the imaginary divine appearances to the mental consciousness such that, although objects continue to appear to the senses, they are no longer ascertained.

Adhering to an attitude of divine pride seems to run contrary to the central Buddhist teaching of selflessness, which is that the inherently existent I, innately conceived to exist by ordinary, ignorant awarenesses, is utterly non-existent. That is, while there is a nominally existent I, there is no inherently existent I even though such an I is naturally conceived to exist. However, divine pride is cultivated only after meditation on emptiness, which negates the false conception of I; hence, the I of deity yoga is not conceived to inherently exist, as is the ordinary I, but rather is understood to be only nominally existent, even when one is completely focused on the thought that one is the deity. Thus, divine pride can actually serve as an *antidote* to the ordinary conception of I and the afflictive pride based on that.[105] Also, this indicates that divine pride is not a wrong consciousness★ — an awareness mistaken with regard to the object it engages — for one creates it deliberately within the context of a practice of imagination. Divine pride is not merely self-delusion, but is an extremely effective fabrication that allows tantric actors to gain liberating insight about themselves through the process of immersing themselves in their roles.

5 Distinguishing Persons from Paths

In the stage of generation, one pretends through creative visualization both that the winds that go out from the sense-powers are being drawn into the body and that those winds and the winds that course through the body are entering, remaining, and dissolving in the central channel. In the stage of completion one no longer merely pretends that the winds are being drawn into the central channel; this process actually occurs. However, there are exceptional cases in which someone practicing the subtle stage of generation, without having begun the specific practices of the stage of completion, experiences the entrance and dissolution of winds in the central channel. Even though these experiences occur to someone of the stage of generation, they are counted as instances of the stage of completion.[106]

Thus, a distinction is made between persons who are *of* the stage of generation and the *paths* they are practicing, which may be designated as sutra paths, paths of the lower tantra sets, or even stage of completion paths, depending upon their activity and/or the effect which results from them. There is nothing extraordinary about the fact that persons of the stage of generation practice sutra paths, for the cultivation of compassion and the realization of emptiness are as essential to tantric practice as they are to sutra practice. It is also not uncommon that such persons practice paths of the lower tantras. It *is* unusual that persons of the stage of generation are said to practice paths of the stage of completion, but there are two instances in which this occurs: (1) at the end of the stage of generation and (2) when an external "seal"* (sexual consort) is used.

In the first case, a spontaneous entry of winds into the central channel may be experienced upon finishing the stage of generation. According to Dzong-ka-ba, the stage of generation is finished at the point where there has been full development of a meditative stabilization that is a union of calm abiding and special insight.

The second instance in which persons not of the stage of completion experience a *path* of the stage of completion can occur when yogis ritually engage in sexual union with consorts called "Knowledge Women"* while vividly imagining that they and their partners are specific deities.[107] By this means, yogis already skilled in meditation on emptiness can mix their realization of emptiness with bliss, turning it into a blissful consciousness realizing emptiness. This blissful consciousness is a path of the stage of completion. (Because that consciousness stamps or seals with bliss all the phenomena that appear to it, the consort who helps to induce it is called a "seal".[108]) Persons who use this method, which is normally reserved for practices of the stage of completion, are still considered to be of the stage of generation because they have not perfected their ability in visualization to the point of being able to cause the winds to enter the central channel merely by the power of meditation.

In short, although these persons have finished the stage of generation and are experiencing a path of the stage of completion, Nga-wang-bel-den, following Dzong-ka-ba, calls them persons of the stage of generation rather than persons of the stage of completion.[109] That is because for them the winds do not enter, remain, and dissolve in the central channel due to the power of penetrative focusing on important places in the central channel. Similarly, it is possible to experience the four joys★ — bliss consciousnesses that, on the stage of completion, occur due to the entry, abiding, and dissolution of winds in the central channel — even by receiving initiation,[110] but persons who experience the four joys due to initiation are not considered practitioners of the stage of completion.

Chart 4. *General System of Highest Yoga Tantra*

Stages	Levels of Stages	Dissolution of Winds in Central Channel	Correlation With Sutra Paths
Buddhahood	Non-learner's Union (Buddhahood)		Path of No More Learning
Stage of Completion	Learner's Union	At Indestructible Drop at Heart (all winds)	Path of Meditation
	Actual Clear Light		Path of Seeing
	Impure Illusory Body		Path of Preparation
	Mental Isolation	At Indestructible Drop at Heart (some winds)	Path of Preparation
	Verbal Isolation	At Heart	
	Physical Isolation	At Lower Opening	
Stage of Generation	Subtle Stage of Generation	Imaginary Dissolution	Path of Accumulation
	Coarse Stage of Generation		

*Solid lines = distinct categories, broken lines = overlapping or equivalent categories.

(read from bottom up)

Part Three
The Stage of Completion
of Highest Yoga Tantra

The Six Levels of the Stage of Completion

The definition of the stage of completion is:[111]

> a yoga in the continuum of a learner that arises from having caused the winds to enter, abide, and dissolve into the central channel by the power of meditation.

In the stage of completion, one is actually transformed into the deity one has merely imagined on the stage of generation. Within the vivid visualization of oneself as a deity and one's environment as divine, one practices penetrative focusing on important points of the body, causing the currents of energy (winds) that course through the body to enter and dissolve in the central channel and then into the indestructible drop in the center of the heart. Using the very subtle and powerful mind of "clear light" that dawns as a result of the total dissolution of winds in the indestructible drop, one realizes emptiness. Rising up in the form of a deity in an illusory body — a body made of wind — and meditating on emptiness with a mind of clear light, one swiftly amasses the collections of wisdom and method, overcomes all of the obstructions to liberation and omniscience, and achieves the final rank of Buddhahood.

There are two principal ways to distinguish the various levels of the stage of completion: by results and by techniques. In other words, separate levels are posited in accordance with the occurrence of actual physical changes that result from the use of special techniques, or else they are distinguished according to the techniques themselves. Nga-wang-bel-den uses the mode of division based on results, mentioning the division by way of techniques only in passing; Part Three of this book is, therefore, set forth in terms of the mode of division based on results.

According to the method of distinguishing the levels of the stage of completion according to results, the six levels of the stage of completion are:

1 physical isolation★
2 verbal isolation★
3 mental isolation★
4 illusory body★
5 actual clear light★
6 learner's union★

Not all presentations of the *Guhyasamāja* system enumerate the levels in this manner; some others condense the first two or the first three levels into a single level (but do not make any other changes in the mode of positing levels or determining their limits).[112] Also, physical isolation, the first level of the stage of completion, is considered to be a yoga of both the stage of generation and the stage of completion.[113] Nga-wang-bel-den implies this since his definition of physical isolation specifies that it is the physical isolation *which is a stage of completion*, suggesting that there is also a physical isolation of the stage of generation, this being preparatory to the actual dissolution of winds in the central channel.

When the levels of the stage of completion are distinguished by way of techniques, there are also six:[114]

1 withdrawal★

2 concentration*
3 lengthening vitality and exertion*
4 retention*
5 subsequent mindfulness*
6 meditative stabilization*

1 Physical Isolation

The definition of physical isolation is:[115]

> that stage of completion ranging from the point at
> which a yogi who has completed the subtle stage of
> generation of this system, through meditation on
> [the entire mandala in a] subtle [drop] at the lower
> opening, produces an exalted wisdom of emptiness
> that arises through the winds entering, abiding, and
> dissolving in the central channel, through to but not
> including generating the exalted wisdom that arises
> from the upper and lower winds dissolving in the
> central channel at the heart.

The meditation on a mandala in a subtle drop is the main
practice of the subtle stage of generation of this Highest
Yoga Tantra system. In the stage of generation, the drop is
clearly visualized at either the upper or lower opening of the
central channel; here, in the stage of completion, it is
visualized only at the lower opening (the tip of the sexual
organ). This subtle drop, though extremely tiny, is to be
seen as containing the entire mandala, with deities, palace,
guards, and so forth. Because immense concentration is
required to generate this extremely subtle product of im-

agination, when it is actualized the accompanying mental concentration pulls the winds back from sense objects and draws them to the lower opening of the central channel, where the subtle mandala is being visualized.

When this subtle drop yoga actually causes some of the winds to enter, remain, and dissolve in the central channel at the lower opening (which in turn causes the manifestation of subtler consciousnesses called "empties", which will be explained below), it then technically fulfills the definition of the yoga of physical isolation of the stage of completion. During the meditative practices associated with this level, the winds enter the central channel, and some of the channel-knots begin to loosen, allowing the winds to move in the central channel. Physical isolation is insufficient, however, to loosen the heart channel-knot, which is more difficult to loosen than any other knot, or for causing the winds to be gathered at the heart.[116] The level of physical isolation culminates with the beginning of the loosening of the channel-knot at the heart.

Etymology of Physical Isolation

In tantric practice, the conception and appearance of ordinariness are to be "isolated", i.e., suppressed, in order to protect the mind from them. This does not entail just a withdrawal of the mind from ordinary appearances. The senses are indeed withdrawn from external objects during meditative equipoise in the various levels of the stage of completion, isolating the yogi from the conception and appearance of ordinariness, but withdrawal of old appearances is followed by substitution. One makes ideal substitutions for ordinary appearances by seeing them either as manifestations of bliss and emptiness or as deities. Mere withdrawal of the mind from external objects would not be deity yoga.

The term "physical" in "physical isolation" refers to a meditation practice of this level wherein one views, as deities and a divine environment, the twenty types of gross objects (consisting of the five aggregates, the four constituents, the six sources, and five objects)[117] which comprise all impermanent phenomena. One is thus "isolated" from the appearance of the physical world as ordinary.

Neither "isolation" nor "physical" is exclusive to the level of physical isolation. All levels of the stage of completion and the stage of generation are isolations because they suppress the conception and appearance of ordinariness. Moreover, the visualization of all phenomena as deities and a divine environment, the so-called "physical isolation", is carried out at all levels of both stages. However, here those terms serve to demarcate the initial level of the stage of completion.

Divisions of Physical Isolation

The two major divisions of physical isolation are (1) withdrawal and (2) concentration. Concentration is further divided into five parts: (i) individual investigation, (ii) analysis, (iii) mental bliss, (iv) bliss of pliancy, and (v) meditative stabilization of a one-pointed mind. These parts are not, however, practiced in the order listed; mental bliss, bliss of pliancy, and meditative stabilization are actually performed first, because they are facets of meditative equipoise, whereas withdrawal, individual investigation, and analysis are activities performed subsequent to meditation. Moreover, these divisions are clearly not exhaustive because the description of the practice of the level of physical isolation suggests that all six of the divisions and sub-divisions are associated only with the second, third, and fourth phases of a four-phase process of meditation,[118] on which the following discussion is based.

The four distinct phases of meditation in the level of physical isolation are: (1) meditation on a subtle drop; (2) meditation on emptiness using a mind embued with bliss; (3) meditation in which one views everything that appears as a manifestation of bliss and emptiness; and (4) returning to meditative equipoise on emptiness.

Meditation on a Subtle Drop

As explained earlier, the meditation on a subtle drop in the level of physical isolation is essentially the continuation of the meditation on a subtle drop performed in the subtle stage of generation. The entire mandala of deities and a divine mansion, containing representatives of all types of objects, is visualized in a subtle (tiny) drop at the lower opening of the central channel (the tip of the sexual organ).[119] Due to intense concentration on that point, the winds are drawn to the lower opening of the central channel and begin to enter the central channel there. This causes the downward-voiding wind, whose seat is in the lower abdomen, to turn upwards, igniting the heat of the Fierce Woman*,[120] which in turn melts some of the white drop and causes the manifestation of the four joys and four empties. Before continuing with the description of the other phases of meditation in the level of physical isolation, the "Fierce Woman", white and red drops, four empties, and four joys will be explained further.

Fierce Woman. "Fierce Woman" is the literal translation of *gtu mo*, the name of the heat yogis generate in the abdominal region through intense concentration. Yogic techniques to ignite heat are indispensible to tantric practice because they cause the white and red drops — subtle substances that coat the inside of the channels — to melt and flow to various spots, bringing about an intense feeling of bliss; the resulting bliss consciousnesses are powerful awarenesses that can be used to realize emptiness. The bliss engendered by causing the white and red drops to flow in the central channel is said to be a hundred times greater than the pleasure of ordinary orgasm.[121] (In ordinary male orgasm, the white drop is caused to melt and flow near the central channel, its proximity to the central channel being the source of the experience of pleasure.[122] Such orgasmic pleasure is limited because the Fierce Woman is ignited only momentarily, the winds do not flow in the central channel, and the white drop merely passes near the central channel, not within it.)

Causing the Fierce Woman to blaze up is a practice common to all tantras. In *Guhyasamāja*, the Fierce Woman is ignited by wind yoga, but the yoga itself is not called Fierce Woman yoga, or heat yoga, as in some other systems.

The White and Red Drops. The white and red drops, along with the winds and channels, are an integral part of tantric physiology. They are described as the pure essence of the essential fluids of the male and female, having evolved from the original white drop of the father and red drop of the mother that combined to become the original physical basis for the human body at the time of conception.[123] Hence, both the white and red drops are found everywhere in all male and female bodies, where they coat the inside of the channels "like frost."[124] However, the drops are not equally distributed throughout the body, for the white drop predominates at the top of the head and the red predominates at the solar plexus.

The origin of the drops is the "indestructible drop" at the heart, a tiny drop the size of a large mustard seed or small pea, with a white top and red bottom;[125] it is called "indestructible" because the continuum of the very subtle wind within it is never broken.[126] The indestructible drop is actually *two* indestructible drops: (1) the "eternal" indestructible drop, which is the very subtle wind and mind, and (2) the lifetime indestructible drop, which is a subtle material object and is destroyed at the end of an individual's lifetime. The "eternal" drop, which lasts until Buddhahood, is located inside the lifetime drop. Winds dissolve into the lifetime drop and then into the "eternal" drop.[127] The white and red drops located inside the indestructible drop are subtle drops whereas those located in the channels are coarse drops.[128]

When the winds enter, abide, and dissolve in the central channel, thereby causing the Fierce Woman to ignite and melt the white drop, the four empties, the four joys of descent from above, and the four joys of descent from below are generated.

The Four Empties. The entry, abiding, and dissolution of the winds in the central channel generates an "exalted wisdom of emptiness"*. In this context, an exalted wisdom of emptiness is *not* an exalted wisdom consciousness that directly realizes a phenomenon's absence of inherent existence, as these terms suggest. Rather, here an exalted wisdom of emptiness is any one of four subtle minds called "the four empties". These subtle types of consciousness are to be *used* to realize emptiness, but they are not themselves emptinesses nor realizations of emptiness.

The four empties are associated with the entry and dissolution of winds in the central channel. They are the last four of the "signs" accompanying the dissolution of winds (see chart 5). Because these signs are associated with the dissolution of winds in the central channel, they occur not only due to tantric practice, but also in the process of ordinary death, and at the times of going to sleep, experiencing orgasm, and fainting, occasions when winds are drawn into the central channel. At all of those times, each of the signs in chart 5 (p. 74) appear to the mind.

The four empties are respectively termed "the empty", "the very empty", "the great empty", and "the all-empty" and are also called the mind of radiant white appearance*, the mind of radiant red or orange increase*, the mind of radiant black near-attainment*, and the mind of clear light*. The first empty, the mind of white appearance, is brought about when, because all the winds from the right and left channels enter into the central channel above the heart, the white drop* located at the top of the head melts and drips down to the top of the heart. (Drops will be explained in a later section). When the drop arrives at the top of the heart, the mind is filled with a brilliant white

Chart 5. *Signs Accompanying Dissolutions*

Dissolution	Sign or Appearance to Mind
1 Winds Enter Central Channel	Equal Breath in Both Nostrils
2 Winds Remain in Central Channel	No Movement of Air in Nostrils
3 Earth Element Dissolves Into Water Element	Appearance Like Mirage
4 Water Element Dissolves Into Fire Element	Appearance Like Smoke
5 Fire Element Dissolves Into Wind Element	Appearance Like Fireflies
6 Wind Element Dissolves Into Consciousness	Appearance Like Butter-lamp Flickering, Then Steady
7 Eighty Indicative Conceptions Dissolve Into White Appearance	Appearance Like Moonlight in Clear Autumn Sky
8 White Appearance Dissolves Into Red/Orange Increase	Appearance Like Sunlight in Clear Autumn Sky
9 Red Increase Dissolves Into Black Near-Attainment	Appearance Like Thick Blackness in Clear Autumn Night Sky
10 Black Near-Attainment Dissolves Into Clear Light	Appearance Like Natural Color of a Clear Autumn Dawn Sky

light like moonlight, whereby it gets the name radiant white appearance.[129]

This mind full of white light is also called "the empty" because it is devoid of the "eighty indicative conceptions"* and the coarse winds that serve as their mount. The eighty indicative conceptions are the eighty types of conceptual consciousnesses — ordinary minds such as sorrow or happiness that get at their objects indirectly by way of a generic image*.[130] These are simply the wholesome and unwholesome conceptual awarenesses of ordinary experience, ranging from hatred to compassion.[131] The four subtle minds of white appearance, red or orange increase, black near-attainment, and clear light are thus devoid of all coarse conceptuality, but the first three of these are nevertheless said to be conceptual consciousnesses because they are neither devoid of subject-object duality nor of the appearance of inherent existence.

The second empty, the mind of red or orange increase, occurs when the winds in the right and left channels *below* the heart have entered the central channel through the lower opening, causing the red drop located at the navel to ascend toward the heart. When the red drop touches the lower part of the channel-knot at the heart, the mind is filled with a reddish appearance like sunlight. It is called "very empty" because it is devoid not only of all the coarse winds, but even of the mind of white appearance and the wind that is its mount.

The third empty, the mind of black near-attainment, occurs when, through the force of the winds being gathered at the heart, the heart channel-knot is loosened, enabling the white drop above the heart and the red drop below the heart to move to the indestructible drop in the center of the heart. When the white and red drops meet, the mind is filled with a vacuous blackness like a clear autumn night sky.[132] One eventually swoons into unconsciousness. This mind is called "near-attainment" because of its proximity to the mind of clear light and is called "great empty" because of being devoid not only of all the coarse winds, but even of the mind of red increase and the wind that is its mount.

The fourth empty, the mind of clear light, is the most subtle consciousness possible. It occurs when all of the winds dissolve into the very subtle vitalizing wind and the red and white drops are dissolved into the red and white parts of the indestructible drop. At that time the very subtle primordial wind and mind of clear light become manifest* and the mind is filled with a totally non-dualistic appearance of a mere vacuity free from the white, red, and black appearances. The mind of clear light is called the "all-empty" because it is completely devoid of all other subtle and coarse minds and winds.

The four empties cannot occur until winds have entered, remained, and dissolved in the central channel; hence, the four empties are merely imaginary on the stage of generation and are not fully-qualified on the stage of completion until the end of the level of mental isolation.

Again, the empties should not be confused with emptinesses, the absences of inherent existence of persons and all other phenomena. The empties are subtle consciousnesses which are used to *realize* emptiness. They occur whenever winds enter the central channel, such as at the time of death, when going to sleep, fainting, and orgasm. They can be used by highly skilled yogis not only when they are brought about by the techniques of the stage of completion, but also at the times when they naturally occur.[133] However, making use of them at such times is extremely difficult. For instance, even though the mind of clear light of the ordinary process of death can be used to realize emptiness, dying persons are typically engrossed in the terror of annihilation and are thus unable to make use of that mind for any purpose.[134]

The Four Joys. The four joys[135] are bliss consciousnesses generated because of the melting of the drop and its movement in the central channel.[136] In order of least to greatest, they are called joy*, supreme joy*, special joy*, and innate joy*. There are various other ways of distinguishing the joys. For instance, in the context of physical isolation, the joys generated by the descent of the drop from the top of the head are distinguished from those generated by the ascent of the drop from the "secret place" at the base of the spine. The joys generated from the ascent of the drop are much more powerful than those generated from the descent of the drop; all of the joys from the ascent of the drop are considered innate joys, the type with the greatest intensity.

Thus, although there are said to be four joys from above and four joys from below, the joys from above and from below are not necessarily the four — joy, supreme joy, special joy, and innate joy — since the four from below are all innate joys. Rather, the four joys above and below are posited not according to the intensity of bliss, but according to the movement of the drops in the central channel. The four joys from above are generated respectively when the white drop flows down from the crown to the throat, from there to the heart, from there to the navel, and from there to the base of the spine.[137] The four joys from below are generated respectively when the red drop rises from the base of the spine to the navel, from there to the heart, from there to the throat, and from there to the crown.

On the path, when the four joys are produced as a result of the entry and dissolution of winds in the central channel, they are also often called the four empties. Many scholars follow the explanation that the four joys simply *are* the four empties. Their assumption probably is that the empties — subtle consciousnesses that occur when the winds are withdrawn — and the joys — subtle bliss consciousnesses that occur when the winds are withdrawn — are in fact the same consciousnesses described from different perspectives. Nga-wang-bel-den disagrees, citing Dzong-ka-ba's refusal to equate the four empties and the four joys, as well as Dzong-ka-ba's approval of the explanation by Tup-ba-bel (*thub pa dpal*) that the four empties are also generated during the white drop's traversal of the sexual organ.[138] Moreover, the four empties could not be identical to the four joys simply because at the time of death there is no experience of the joys whereas there is experience of the empties.

Meditation on Emptiness with Bliss
In the first phase of meditation on the level of physical
isolation, one visualized the subtle drop filled with the array
of visualized deities and the divine mansion; this caused the
winds to enter, remain, and dissolve in the central channel,
the Fierce Woman to be ignited, the drops to flow, and
great bliss to be engendered. Now, once that has occurred,
one is to associate the four joys and emptiness as subject and
object in meditative equipoise. In other words, one is to use
the blissful consciousness that has been created to realize
emptiness.

At this point in the meditation, one begins to practice the
aspects of physical isolation called mental bliss, bliss of
pliancy, and the one-pointed meditative stabilization, three
different aspects of one consciousness meditating on emptiness within the force of great bliss. (These aspects are not
distinguished with precision in Nga-wang-bel-den's text.)
Deities do not appear to this bliss consciousness, but because it is generated due to much previous visualization of
deities, its three aspects of bliss, pliancy, and meditative
stabilization are still considered instances of deity yoga. For
the same reason, even though those three aspects would not
fit the etymology of physical isolation because they do not
involve isolation from ordinary appearances by substituting
ideal appearances, they are still considered physical isolations.

Viewing Appearances As Bliss and Emptiness
After having used the bliss consciousness to realize emptiness, it is said that one should remember bliss and emptiness, restraining all other mental activities so that whatever
appears seems to be a manifestation of bliss and emptiness.
As Dzong-ka-ba says:[139]

> An internal object — a special physical tangible
> object — is produced through melting the mind of
> enlightenment by means of a method of penetrative

focusing on important places on and in the body. That serves as the observed-object condition* whereby a special blissful feeling of the body consciousness is generated. That [special blissful feeling] acts as an immediately preceding condition* whereby the mental consciousness is generated as an entity of marvelous bliss. At that time, through remembering the meaning of suchness that has already been ascertained, emptiness and bliss are associated.

The dripping of the white drop in the central channel produces an extraordinarily blissful body consciousness, which in turn produces a blissful mental consciousness. Then, with the recollection of emptiness, bliss and emptiness are associated.

The restraint of other mental activities so that everything will appear to be a manifestation of bliss and emptiness is the practice of withdrawal, probably so-called because manifestations of bliss and emptiness appear to the sixth consciousness, the mental consciousness, dominating the sense consciousnesses and causing them to withdraw. Through withdrawal, one's mind is so permeated with a feeling of bliss that all appearances are strongly affected. Concurrently, recollection of meditation on emptiness makes phenomena appear to be light, ephemeral, and like illusions. Everything appears to be "sealed" with bliss and emptiness.

This type of imagination is a similitude of a Buddha's actual mode of perceiving phenomena at all times. To Buddhas, phenomena are always sealed with bliss and emptiness. This means that there is a sense in which a consciousness viewing the world as sealed with bliss and emptiness is not faulty, not contradicted by valid cognition.[140]

The practice of withdrawal is essentially a matter of continuing a visualization begun on the stage of generation, when one imagined the world to be a manifestation of bliss and emptiness. However, the same practice on the stage of completion is much more powerful due to the force of one's experience, the immense infusion of bliss that one has experienced as a result of wind and heat yogas.

There are two, more difficult, variations on the practice of withdrawal, one called "individual investigation" and the other called "analysis". In individual investigation, one mentally divides all of the phenomena of the world into the twenty types of gross objects, and then sees them all not only as manifestations of bliss and emptiness, but as taking on either the specific form of a single deity, Vajradhara, or the forms of five deities. It is called investigation because it investigates the entity of the deity inasmuch as it sees that the deity is an expression of bliss and emptiness. One pretends that the mind realizing emptiness appears as the twenty types of gross objects, which in turn appear as either Vajradhara or as five deities.[141]

"Analysis" is similar to individual investigation but is much more demanding. In analysis, one mentally divides the twenty gross objects into one hundred objects and then visualizes them as twenty deities each of which have five lineages (of the Buddhas Vairochana, Akṣhobhya, Amoghasiddhi, Amitābha, and Ratnasambhava).[142] The practice is called "analysis" because it analyzes in detail the specific features of the deities.

Deities. The deities which are vividly visualized in tantric meditation are the imagined forms of various Buddhas who appear either as Buddhas or as Bodhisattvas of high rank.[143] Bodhisattvas are beings who have generated the altruistic aspiration to attain Buddhahood for the welfare of others. Those of high rank are well advanced on the Bodhisattva grounds, which is to say that they have acquired many of the abilities of Buddhas though not in the full measure of Buddhas. Since it is recognized that both Buddhas and high rank Bodhisattvas have the ability to emanate to sentient beings in any manner that will be helpful, even as ordinary objects that people unthinkingly pass over in their daily routines, it is permissible to imagine these enlightened beings in any conceivable form.

However, in practice, tantric manuals prescribe a certain number of deities (for instance, thirty-two in *Guhyasamāja*) and describe them in varying degrees of detail. The purpose of those descriptions is to assist the meditator, who must attempt to construct a mental picture of the mandala for visualization practice, although such a person will probably also be assisted by a painting (such as the Tibetan tang-ga [*thang ka*]) which has been drawn and colored to match the description.

A tantra is usually named after its principal deity. The tantra that is the basis for Nga-wang-bel-den's text, the *Guhyasamāja Tantra*, has Guhyasamāja, one of the many emanated forms of the Buddha Akṣhobhya, as its principal deity. Although there are thirty-two deities in the mandala, they are all, in fact, held to be emanations of Guhyasamāja.[144] In a detailed manual for the practice of a particular tantra — its "means of achievement" — there would be a precise depiction of the position, posture, color, ornaments, and so forth, of Guhyasamāja, his consort, and the other deities in the *Guhyasamāja* mandala, as well as all the features of their environment.

The manual also sometimes contains a lengthy discussion of the symbolic significance of all the details mentioned in the description, aimed at enhancing one's development of divine pride, the sense that one actually *is* the deity one imagines. For instance, in the water initiation portion of the *Kālachakra* initiations for the stage of generation, the manual correlates the five seed syllables of the mantra to the five symbols into which they are transformed, five deities with their consorts, the deities that appear on their crowns, and the elements, such as space, wind, and fire, that are cleansed.[145]

Some deities are depicted as being peaceful whereas others are shown to be fierce. In both cases, the tantric iconography symbolizes a union of bliss and emptiness. For example, the fierce deity Chakrasaṃvara holds a skull filled with blood, but the skull symbolizes bliss (because bliss is experienced when the white drop at the crown of the head is melted) and the blood symbolizes the mind realizing emptiness.[146]

The deities imagined in meditation are, in one sense, recognized to be products of the imagination; hence, yogis engaged in deity yoga do not have wrong consciousnesses, i.e., awarenesses, such as an eye consciousness mistaking a distant pillar for a man, that are incorrect with regard to their main object. Even though yogis cultivate "divine pride", a sense of actually being the deity, theirs are not considered a wrong consciousnesses because divine pride is developed deliberately with a high intention.

On the other hand, the deities imagined in meditation are definitely held to exist in fact, for the actual deity is "invited" to enter the imagined deity. There is a seeming paradox in the fact that one is training to become a deity that already has a separate existence, but in fact, the paradox does not exist if it is understood that all Buddhas can take any form, that no form is exclusive. Although one cannot have the same mental continuum as someone who has already become a Buddha, there is no limit to the number of beings who, upon becoming Buddhas, can manifest the form of that Buddha. Thus, according to the Ge-luk-ba presentation, at least one prominent Buddhist scholar is clearly mistaken when he claims that the images of deities have no reality whatsoever and are abandoned by becoming aware of one's "bodhi-essence".[147]

Deities are visualized in a mandala, a symbolic representation of a divine mansion and its immediate environment in which the principal deity and his consort are at the center. As mentioned above, each tantra has its own particular mandala which is often represented in paintings or carvings in two dimensions, as seen from above, with the tops of its walls and porticos pointing out to the sides.

Returning to Meditation on Emptiness

In the previous three phases of meditation — meditation on a subtle drop; meditation on emptiness with bliss; and meditation viewing appearances as bliss and emptiness — one meditated on a subtle drop at the lower opening of the central channel, used the resulting bliss consciousness to meditate on emptiness, and emerged from meditative equipoise, seeing all phenomena as a manifestation of bliss and emptiness. In the fourth phase of meditation, one is drawn back into meditative equipoise because bliss has caused the winds of the sense powers to withdraw inside. This in turn increases bliss because the winds ignite the Fierce Woman, which melts the drops, causing them to flow in the central channel, producing great bliss.

The way in which meditation leads to bliss and bliss draws one back into meditative equipoise illustrates one of the great differences between the paths of tantra and the paths of sutra. Once one has gained facility in the very formidable visualization practices of tantra and has had success in meditation on emptiness, the tantric path gets easier rather than more difficult; bliss and meditation on emptiness become mutually supportive. One meditates on emptiness with a mind empowered with bliss; then, subsequent to meditative equipoise, one sees everything as bliss, which causes the sense powers to withdraw, the Fierce Woman to ignite, the drops to flow, and bliss to increase, drawing one back into meditative equipoise on emptiness. This cycle occurs again and again. Moreover, just seeing phenomena as manifestations of bliss helps one to realize their lack of inherent existence, their emptiness. As the Dalai Lama has said, when phenomena appear to be the sport or manifestation of the mind of clear light one can understand all the better that they are empty and just nominally designated.[148]

2 Verbal Isolation

The definition of verbal isolation is:[149]

> a stage of completion that is a state beginning from
> the point at which a yogi of this system generates
> the exalted wisdom of appearance that arises from
> the three — the winds of the upper and lower
> openings entering, remaining, and dissolving into
> the central channel at the heart due to having medi-
> tated on a mantra drop at the point of the heart. It
> ranges up to but does not include having generated
> the exalted wisdom of appearance which arises from
> the winds entering, abiding, and dissolving into the
> indestructible drop at the heart upon loosening
> completely the channel-knot at the heart by the
> power of meditation.

On the level of verbal isolation, winds are caused to enter,
remain, and dissolve into the central channel at the heart
but have not yet entered, remained, and dissolved in the
indestructible drop in the center of the heart.

Etymology of Verbal Isolation
Although physical isolation involves the substitution of

divine appearances for ordinary appearances, verbal isolation does not similarly involve the substitution of divine speech for ordinary language. It is true that "speech" is to be isolated, but here "speech" refers not to verbal communication but rather to the three phases of the activity of breathing: (1) inhalation, (2) the pause before exhalation when the breath is held, and (3) exhalation. What is to be isolated, that is, suppressed, is the ordinary worldly conception about these three phases of breathing, namely, that their "tones" are not identical with the "tones" of the three letters, OM, ĀH, and HŪM. In fact, says Nga-wang-belden, the "tones" of the three phases of breathing, the breath's natural reverberations which occur every moment but ordinarily escape notice, *are* identical with OM, ĀH, and HŪM.

The practice of verbal isolation, therefore, is to *notice* that the natural reverberation of the breath sounds like OM, ĀH, and HŪM. This means that one is to realize only that the reverberation of the three phases of breathing when the winds move in the central channel are the tones of OM, ĀH, and HŪM, not to think that these reverberations are identical with the written letters OM, ĀH, and HŪM, nor that they are identical with the external vocalizing of these syllables, nor that they are identical with the mental recollection of such external vocalization.[150]

The level of verbal isolation is named after the second of its three yogas, the meditation on a light drop at the point of the nose, during which the actual verbal isolation takes place. The first and third yogas of the level of verbal isolation — the meditation on the mantra drop at the heart and the meditation on the substance drop at the sexual organ — are designated as verbal isolation but are not actual verbal isolation because they do not actually involve the association of the breath with certain syllables.

The yoga of the level of verbal isolation is one that is manifestly concerned with the breath, and hence is a "lengthening of vitality"* (i.e., breath) yoga (*prāṇāyāma*). It is only one of several types of tantric wind yogas, some of which have already been discussed. *Prāṇāyāma* is a very broad term; it includes all meditations — on letters, drops, and so forth — that gather winds in the central channel. In *Kālachakra* and in the lower tantras, *prāṇāyāma* means *restraint* of the winds, but in the *Guhyasamāja Tantra prāṇāyāma* also comes to mean "lengthening of vitality" in the sense that the central channel, ordinarily empty, is being filled with winds. There is also a lengthening of vitality in the sense of longer life; humans are said to be limited to 21,600 breaths per day over the lifespan determined by their particular karma, and vitality-lengthening yoga expands the lifespan by causing the rate of breathing to be slowed.[151]

Meditation on a Mantra Drop

Verbal isolation comprises three wind yogas that utilize three different types of subtle drops: the mantra drop⋆, the light drop⋆, and the substance drop⋆.[152] The first yoga of verbal isolation is a meditation on a "mantra" drop — a drop the nature of which is imagined to be the mantra syllable HŪṂ — imagined at the heart channel-wheel in the shape of the Tibetan punctuation mark, the shay (*shad*),[153] which resembles a spike, thick at the top and tapering to the bottom. (This means that the mantra drop looks like a shay, not like the syllable HŪṂ, even though it is imagined that its nature is HŪṂ.) As a result of focusing on this point, winds from both the upper and lower parts of the body are drawn into the central channel and thence into the area of the heart. The entry and dissolution of winds there in turn brings about at least the first of the four empties, the mind of radiant white appearance in which the mind is absorbed in an appearance which is like brilliant white moonlight. The production of the first empty marks the actual beginning of the level of verbal isolation.[154] Even though the winds have dissolved in the central channel at the heart, at this stage the channel-knots at the heart are still tight, preventing the winds from moving.

Meditation on a Light Drop

The second yoga of verbal isolation, meditation on the light drop, actually causes the winds to enter, remain, and dissolve into the indestructible drop in the center of the heart. One meditates on a drop of light imagined to be at the point of the nose. This drop is called a light drop because it is very clear, imagined as if it had a nature of light.[155] As the breath is imagined to pass by this drop of light, one is simply to observe that it reverberates with the sounds OM, ĀḤ, and HŪṂ in the phases of inhalation, retention, and exhalation, respectively. This observation, also called "vajra repetition"*, enables the winds in the central channel to move back and forth and forces the knots to loosen a little.[156] When, due to that, the winds begin to enter, remain, and dissolve into the indestructible drop, producing the first empty, the level of verbal isolation ends and the level of mental isolation begins.

After some success has been gained in the light drop yoga, one switches from observation of the four basic winds to observation of the five secondary winds. The basic winds are the ordinary five winds with the exception of the pervasive wind; thus, the four basic winds are the vitalizing, fire-accompanying, downward-voiding, and upward-moving winds, associated respectively with water, fire, earth, and wind.[157] The secondary winds are those associated with the senses; they are actually included within the basic winds, being branches of the vitalizing basic wind. By switching one's observation of the breath from the basic winds to the secondary winds, the channel-knots are loosened further and the winds are allowed greater access to the indestructible drop at the heart. Vajra repetition is an important practice of the stage of completion; Nga-wang-bel-den mentions that even though it is not mentioned in connection with subsequent levels, it can be continued right through the level of union.

Meditation on a Substance Drop

The third yoga of verbal isolation, the meditation on the substance drop, enhances the process of drawing winds into the indestructible drop. The substance drop is imagined to be composed of the white and red drops; in the meditation on it, one imagines a drop at the point where there is a meeting of the two lower openings of the two central channels of oneself and either a real or imagined "seal" (a sexual consort that assists one to achieve a bliss consciousness that realizes emptiness, "sealing" phenomena with bliss and emptiness).[158] This sexual union, real or imagined, causes the substance drop to appear at the tip of the sexual organ, but the drop is not emitted, being willfully held in place. The seal with whom one is in sexual union may be either real or imagined. However, if the seal is merely a Wisdom Seal*, an imagined consort, one can attain only the level of mental isolation, not the *final* mental isolation that results in an illusory body in one's present lifetime.[159] An Action Seal*, an actual consort, is needed in order to complete all the qualities of mental isolation, because one needs to withdraw all of the winds just as they are withdrawn at death in order to rise in an illusory body.

This yoga serves to further enhance the loosening of the channel-knots and the collection of winds into the indestructible drop. As will be seen, the definition of the level of mental isolation seems to imply that the substance drop yoga is in fact necessary for the full loosening of the knots.

When the three drop yogas of verbal isolation have caused the dissolution of at least some of the winds in the indestructible drop, one passes to the level of mental isolation.

3 Mental Isolation

The definition of the level of mental isolation is:[160]

> the stage of completion from the point at which one
> generates the exalted wisdom of appearance that has
> arisen due to the dissolution of the winds in the
> indestructible drop at the heart — having fully un-
> tied the channel knot at the heart in dependence
> upon (1) internal conditions, [namely] vajra repeti-
> tion and the stages of withdrawal of the two concen-
> trations, and (2) an external condition, vitality-
> lengthening involving a seal — for as long as one has
> not achieved an impure illusory body.

Mental isolation begins with the manifestation of the
empties due to the dissolution of winds in the indestructible
drop in the heart, and it ends just before one rises in an
illusory body. There are actually two types of mental isolation: a *mere* mental isolation that is achieved by depending
on a Wisdom Seal — an imagined consort — and a *final*
mental isolation that can only be achieved with an Action
Seal — an actual consort — or at death. A final mental
isolation is a prerequisite for passing on to the next level of
the stage of completion, the level of illusory body. Mere

mental isolation requires the dissolution of at least some of the winds into the indestructible drop whereas the final mental isolation occurs only if all of the winds are dissolved in it.

On the level of mental isolation, that which is isolated, or suppressed, is conceptuality; the mind is isolated from conceptuality by being made to appear as an entity of undifferentiable bliss and emptiness.[161] The practices begun on the level of verbal isolation are continued. To proceed from mental isolation to the next level, that of the illusory body, one must switch from an imagined to an actual consort if one has not done so already.

Two Conditions for Attaining Mental Isolation

The internal and external conditions one must depend upon in order to attain the level of mental isolation and bring it to completion are very similar to the practices of the level of verbal isolation. The *internal* condition is vajra repetition — the second yoga of verbal isolation, the actual verbal isolation in which, visualizing a drop of light at the upper opening of the central channel (between the eyebrows), one observes the reverberation of the breath as OM, ĀH, and HŪM — and two stages of "withdrawal" involving visualization practices.[162] The first type of withdrawal involves a visualization in which one imagines a Buddha's Pure Land, marvelous in appearance and filled with deities, and a syllable, HŪM, located at the heart, from which light rays are emitted. The rays of light emitted from the HŪM at one's heart are imagined to dissolve the environment and the beings of the Buddha's Pure Land; the resulting mass of light then dissolves in one's own body, and coalesces into one's heart; after that, appearances cease, and one meditates on emptiness. The second type of withdrawal does not involve the imagination of a Buddha's Pure Land, and so forth. One imagines that the light rays emitted by the HŪM at one's heart dissolve one's body into light; subsequently, appearances cease and one meditates on emptiness.[163]

The *external* condition of mental isolation is either a Wisdom Seal or an Action Seal. The Wisdom Seal is an internal (imagined) seal whereas the Action Seal is an external (actual) seal; thus, it is not the case that the *external* condition of mental isolation must be an *external* seal, in the sense of an actual consort. An Action Seal is a special partner, one who must have received initiation in the tantra, know its meaning, keep the pledges and vows, and at least have experience of the stage of generation, if not the stage of completion. Some tantras even specify the shape, type of eyes, tone of voice, and skills in the sixty-four "arts of love" that should be possessed by an ideal Action Seal.[164]

Certain activities are carried out with an Action Seal to increase bliss and thereby enhance the consciousness that realizes emptiness. These deeds*[165] (see chart 6) are performed after attaining a mere mental isolation, and their enactment helps one to gain, respectively, the illusory body, a learner's union, and a non-learner's union. Without these deeds, which presuppose the assistance of an Action Seal, enlightenment in one lifetime is impossible.

There are three categories of deeds: the elaborative*, the non-elaborative, and the very non-elaborative. Elaborative deeds involve masks, clothing like that of the Seal, and the "call and response" of the imagined deity and Seal. Non-elaborative deeds also use masks and clothing but do not involve the "elaborations" of call and response. Very non-elaborative deeds involve only sexual union with a Wisdom Seal and use of the clear light of sleep without any external elaborations.

Deeds of all three types are performed both on the stage of generation and the stage of completion. After completing both the coarse and subtle levels of the stage of generation, one performs deeds with a Seal to bring about more quickly the attainment of what are called "common feats" (Buddhahood being the "supreme feat"), which include the control of harmful beings, the increase of intelligence and wealth, clairvoyance, and being able to understand a treatise immediately upon reading it.[166] On the stage of completion, deeds are performed for the purpose of enhancing meditation on emptiness.

Chart 6. *Deeds for Enhancement*

Type of Deed	Activity
Elaborative	Masks, Clothing, etc., and Call and Response
Non-Elaborative	Masks, Clothing, etc.
Very Non-Elaborative	Sexual Union with Wisdom Seal and Clear Light of Sleep

The use of an Action Seal is one of two ways to proceed to the level of illusory body. The only other way to rise in an illusory body is to use one's actual death as the means of withdrawing all the winds, practicing vajra repetition as one is dying. (If one is capable of performing it, this practice would result in an illusory body instead of an intermediate state body and in the attainment of enlightenment without again being reborn into a coarse body.) Shākyamuni Buddha, in his last lifetime prior to enlightenment, used an Action Seal, but it is said that although Dzong-ka-ba also became a Buddha, he did not use an Action Seal, becoming enlightened in the intermediate state instead. Dzong-ka-ba did this because he feared his followers would imitate him without being properly prepared, thus hampering instead of enhancing their practices.[167] Some tantric yogis abstain from the use of a consort out of concern that if they are not properly able to use desire in the path they will destroy what they have previously accomplished and fall into a bad migration. Nga-wang-bel-den, however, states that if one uses an Action Seal after having attained mental isolation, one will incur no such faults.

The Four Empties and the Four Joys
In verbal isolation, the four empties and the four joys are

experienced as the result of the entry, abiding, and dissolution of winds into the central channel and the blazing up of the Fierce Woman, which melts the drops and causes them to flow in the central channel, producing the four joys. In mental isolation, the empties and joys occur as a result of the dissolution of the winds into the indestructible drop, a process that is not completed until the final mental isolation.

As in earlier levels of the stage of completion, one does not experience full-fledged manifestation of the four empties at *mere* mental isolation. The four empties cannot be fully qualified until all of the winds are dissolved in the indestructible drop in the way that they are at death, and this occurs at the very end of mental isolation.[168]

4 Impure Illusory Body

The definition of the level of impure illusory body is:[169]

> the stage of completion starting from the actual achievement of a divine body adorned with the major and minor marks, by way of the following. The metaphoric clear light of the final mental isolation has acted as the cooperative condition, and the fundamental wind that serves as its mount has acted as the substantial cause. Also, simultaneously, the mind of near attainment of the reverse process has been established upon the winds moving slightly from the metaphoric clear light of the final mental isolation. It ranges up to but does not include generation of the proximate causes that are the methods [for actualizing] the actual clear light.

In the level of illusory body, one actually takes on the form of a deity. This occurs in the following manner. First, because of the meditations of the level of mental isolation and the use of an Action Seal, all of the winds dissolve in the indestructible drop in the heart. Then, the mind of metaphoric clear light* — the fourth empty — is experienced. When the winds fluctuate slightly, the form of the deity one has been visualizing in previous levels of the stages of generation and completion suddenly materializes. This is the illusory body; made entirely of non-obstructive wind, it shimmers and moves like a mirage. It appears to be exactly like the body of the deity, except that it is white instead of being multi-colored.[170] At the moment of attaining the illusory body, one begins to re-experience the minds that are coarser than the metaphoric clear light of mental isolation; going through a reverse process, one experiences the minds of black near-attainment, red or orange increase, white appearance, and then the sense and conceptual consciousnesses, all the while appearing in an illusory body.

At this level of the stage of completion, the deity body in which one arises is an *impure* illusory body. It is considered to be impure because one has not yet abandoned the afflictive obstructions★, that is, the obstructions to liberation from cyclic existence established by the afflictions of desire, hatred, and ignorance.[171] (It is not until the level of clear light that those afflictions are eliminated; after liberation one's appearance in an illusory body is pure.) An illusory body is so-called because, like a magician's illusion, it is non-obstructive, being made only of wind, and seen only by the yogi and others who also have attained an illusory body.[172] Nevertheless, it bears the complete markings of a Buddha, which consist of thirty-two major and eighty minor features (such as a crown protrusion, elongated ears, dharma-wheel on the palms, and so forth). An illusory body can separate from the coarse body and go where one wishes it to go, but whether or not it must initially rise inside the coarse body is disputed.[173]

The Coarse, the Subtle, and the Very Subtle

Each sentient being has three types of bodies and minds — the coarse, the subtle, and the very subtle[174] (see chart 7). The coarse body is the body of which we are ordinarily aware, composed of the four elements and the substances evolved from them. The subtle body comprises the channels, winds, and drops. The very subtle body is the very subtle fundamental wind in the indestructible drop that serves as the mount of the mind of clear light. The fundamental wind is called "fundamental" because even though it is impermanent, changing moment to moment, its continuum is eternal. Dwelling in the indestructible drop throughout all of one's previous lifetimes, it continues to exist even at Buddhahood,[175] serving as the mount for the very subtle mind of clear light in which a Buddha continuously abides. It is the most subtle wind, more subtle than the winds in the channels that dissolve into it, those in turn being more subtle than the coarse winds (such as the winds of the sense powers) that dissolve into them.

With regard to minds, the coarse minds are the sense consciousnesses; the subtle mind is the conceptual mental consciousness; and the very subtle mind is the mind of clear light that is mounted upon the very subtle fundamental wind. The difference in the subtlety of these minds is said to be like the quality of the subtlety of the mind at the time of being awake (coarse), when dreaming (subtle), and when in a dreamless sleep[176] (very subtle).

In ordinary waking life, only the coarse body and the coarse and subtle minds (the ordinary sense consciousnesses and the mental consciousness) are manifest. However, in the levels of physical, verbal, and mental isolation of the Highest Yoga Tantra stage of completion, the subtle body of channels, winds, and drops, and the subtle minds of the four empties — white appearance, red increase, black near-attainment, and clear light — also become manifest. (The four empties, except for the actual clear light of the level of clear light, are conceptual consciousnesses because they are not non-dualistic, being affected by the appearance of subject and object and by the appearance of their objects as being inherently existent. Hence, they are only subtle minds, not *very* subtle minds.) The very subtle mind — the mind of clear light — becomes manifest only after all the coarse and subtle winds have dissolved into the indestructible drop at the heart. The very subtle body — the very subtle fundamental wind — also becomes manifest only when the coarse and subtle winds dissolve into the indestructible drop. As previously mentioned, it serves as the mount for the mind of actual clear light. The very subtle wind and mind and the coarser winds and minds never operate simultaneously.

Chart 7. *The Coarse, the Subtle, and the Very Subtle*

	Coarse	*Subtle*	*Very Subtle*
Body	Elements and Evolutes	Channels, Subtle Winds, and Drops	Very Subtle Fundamental Wind
Mind	Sense Consciousnesses	Conceptual Mental Consciousness	Mind of Actual Clear Light

For the illusory body to appear, it is necessary that the subtle and coarse bodies be separated, that is, that the coarse body cease to function. Tantric yogis use one of two ways to separate the bodies. One way of separating the bodies is to use death, which always separates the coarse and subtle bodies (and causes the coarse body to be discarded as a useless corpse). Ordinary death can only be used in the path if a yogi has achieved the level of mental isolation and is able to perform practices associated with verbal isolation — vajra repetition and the two stages of withdrawal — while undergoing the process of death. By doing that, the yogi gains control over the winds, causing them to dissolve into the indestructible drop; then when the mind of clear light becomes manifest at the moment of death, he or she can remain within it,[177] subsequently rising in an illusory body instead of an intermediate state body. After rising in an illusory body, the remaining stages of Highest Yoga Tantra can be completed without again being reborn in a coarse body. Dzong-ka-ba himself is said to have attained enlightenment in place of the intermediate state.[178]

The other way to separate the coarse and subtle bodies is through meditation, which is of two types. The first type of meditation is the practice of transference of consciousness*. One of the practices of the tantric system known as the six yogas of Nāropa, it can be used to transfer one's mind into the body of someone who has just died or to gain rebirth in a Highest Pure Land* at the time of death.[179] It involves the ejection of the fundamental wind and mind, in the form of a deity, from the top of the head by means of wind yoga and repeated imagination. However, transference of consciousness merely separates the coarse and subtle bodies without also leading to the attainment of an illusory body.

The second method of using meditation to separate the coarse and subtle bodies is the meditation of final mental isolation, which involves causing the winds to enter and dissolve in the indestructible drop with the assistance of an Action Seal, an actual consort. The use of an Action Seal is a powerful technique for causing the winds to enter the central channel.[180] This technique alone is sufficient, for when all the winds are totally dissolved in the indestructible drop, all the activities of the coarse body cease and the fundamental wind naturally rises into an illusory body.

As was mentioned earlier, once one rises in an illusory body it is possible to separate from the coarse body according to one's wish. If an illusory body initially rises inside the coarse body, it does so at the heart.[181] One may stay outside the coarse body for as long as one is able to remain in the illusion-like meditative equipoise of final mental isolation, that is, a meditative equipoise in which all objects appear to be like illusions. As the meditative equipoise deteriorates, or as one approaches the end of a previously set-up meditation session, the illusory body re-enters the coarse body. The coarse body cannot be utterly abandoned at this level of practice, because the force of the karma that impells it has not been destroyed (and will not be destroyed until the level of actual clear light). However, even later, when one has a *pure* illusory body and no longer needs the coarse body, the coarse body need not be abandoned; if, for the sake of others, it would serve a purpose to continue in one's old form, the old coarse body can become one of one's emanation bodies.

Enlightenment is actually attained in a *pure* illusory body as one passes from a learner's union to the non-learner's union (Buddhahood) and it occurs in the same lifetime that one attains the impure illusory body. It is not possible to become enlightened in the coarse body; hence, Shākyamuni Buddha's attainment of enlightenment under the bodhi tree in India was a display done for the sake of others, his enlightenment having been accomplished prior to his birth as Siddhartha Gautama, prince of the Shākyas. The only sense in which it is possible to achieve enlightenment in one body in one lifetime is when "one body" is taken to mean one *coarse* body, for in tantric practice one initially uses a coarse body but later switches to a very subtle body — the pure illusory body composed of the very subtle fundamental wind — to finish the path.

The Four Empties and the Illusory Body

The illusory body has two causes: the mind of metaphoric clear light of mental isolation and the fundamental wind that serves as its mount. The fundamental wind in the indestructible drop is the "substantial cause"* of the illusory body, the material from which it develops. The mind of metaphoric clear light is, therefore, a "cooperative condition"* of the illusory body; it is a necessary element of the production of the illusory body because the fundamental wind would not be manifest in its absence. The mind of clear light of mental isolation is "metaphoric" because it is not an actual mind of clear light, being tainted by subtle dualistic appearance. (The actual clear light is the non-conceptual, non-dualistic realization of emptiness by a mind of great innate bliss.)

When one initially rises in an illusory body, one reverses out of the mind of clear light that dawned at the end of the

level of mental isolation, going back into the third empty —
black near-attainment — and subsequently into the second
empty, first empty, and eighty indicative conceptions.
These minds are called the empties, etc., of the "reverse"
process because the mind, having gone "forward" through
the minds of white appearance, red increase, black near-
attainment, and clear light as more winds entered and dissolved in the indestructible drop, now reverses the process
as the very subtle fundamental wind takes shape as an
illusory body.

The attainment of the impure illusory body at the beginning of the "reverse" process after having achieved the
metaphoric clear light of mental isolation is similar to the
way an intermediate state body is manifested in the process
of death, intermediate state, and rebirth. At the time of
death, the mind of clear light of death becomes manifest;
immediately after it has ceased, the coarser minds serially
manifest, beginning with the mind of black near-attainment
of the reverse process, and an intermediate state body — a
type of illusory body — instantaneously rises from the
fundamental wind.[182]

Acquiring the ability to manifest an illusory body means,
in effect, that one has overcome death forever. Ordinarily
one has no control over the process of death, intermediate
state, and rebirth, being powerlessly drawn into cyclic existence again and again; but one who has attained an illusory body cannot die, for to die means to experience the
process of death due to the impelling force of karma, thence
to be drawn into an intermediate state body and thence to
be drawn into yet another birth. One who has achieved an
illusory body has gained control over the winds and can
experience the process of death without entering the intermediate state and taking rebirth.

Exemplification of the Illusory Body
The *Illumination of the Texts of Tantra* uses twelve
metaphors to exemplify the illusory body. The illusory

body is likened to:

1 a human emanated by a magician, because it is only wind and mind;[183]
2 the reflection of the moon in water, because just as the moon, reflected in hundreds of puddles, seems to be everywhere, so the illusory body can spontaneously appear anywhere;[184]
3 a shadow, because it is an appearance of a body without flesh and bones;
4 a mirage, because it shimmers and fluctuates;
5 a dream body, because of being mere wind and mind, separate from the coarse or fruitional body (that is, the ordinary coarse body that is the fruit of karma);
6 an echo, because just as an echo seems to be disassociated from the original sound that was its cause, so the illusory body, though actually one continuum with a fruitional body,[185] appears to be different from it;
7 a city of scent-eaters or *fata morgana*, because just as the tiny beings called "scent-eaters" inhabit cities that seem to appear or disappear suddenly, an illusory body instantaneously appears or disappears;[186]
8 a hallucination, because just as many figures can appear in a hallucination, the illusory body can appear to be many;
9 a rainbow, because its colors are unmixed;
10 lightening in dark clouds, because just as lightening flashes within clouds, an illusory body abides in the aggregates of the fruitional body;
11 a water bubble, because just as a water bubble rises up suddenly out of the water, an illusory body arises all at once from emptiness; and
12 a mirror-image of Vajradhara, because all its limbs are complete.

The best of these examples is said to be the dream body because (1) it is the only example that actually is itself a type of illusory body, and (2) its precursor, actuality, and conclusion — that is, what immediately precedes it, what it is, and how it ends — exemplify the illusory body (see chart 8). A dream body is a subtle body made of wind and mind that issues forth out of the coarse body after one has gone to sleep. Even ordinary people have dream bodies, but most have no control over them, whereas yogis can use them to travel about and perform various activities.[187] The dream body is itself an actual illusory body (though not one produced by the path) because it is a body made of wind and mind, either abiding within the coarse body or issuing out of it after the winds have been withdrawn and one has experienced the four empties (very briefly) at the time of sleep.

The precursor, actuality, and conclusion of the dream body exemplify the precursor, actuality, and conclusion of the illusory body as follows. The empties that are always briefly experienced at the time of going to sleep and which are the precursor of the dream body, are similar to the empties experienced on the path that are the precursor of the illusory body. Then, the dream body itself exemplifies the illusory body because it is itself a type of illusory body, being a body made of wind. The conclusion of the dream body is the dream body's return to the coarse body at the end of the dream, which is like the illusory body's return to the coarse body or emanation body.

Chart 8. *The Illusory Body and the Dream Body*

Phase	Exemplifier	Exemplified
Precursor	Empties Experienced Before Sleep	Empties Experienced Before Illusory Body
Actuality	Dream Body	Illusory Body
Conclusion	Dream Body's Return to Coarse Body at End of Dream	Illusory Body's Return to Coarse Body or Emanation Body

In a similar way, the illusory body, mind of clear light, and emanated forms exemplify the three bodies of a Buddha — the Truth Body, Complete Enjoyment Body, and Emanation Body[188] (see chart 9). In reality, a Buddha's Truth Body is the actual clear light, the mind of great innate bliss directly realizing emptiness; his Complete Enjoyment Body is the pure illusory body, the magnificent form body made of the very subtle fundamental wind; and his Emanation Body is the variety of forms he manifests for the sake of sentient beings. On the path of Highest Yoga Tantra,[189] there are similitudes of the three bodies of the Buddha: the actual clear light of the stage of completion is like the Buddha's Truth Body; the impure illusory body is like his Complete Enjoyment Body; and the use of the old coarse body as an emanation body by one who has attained an illusory body is like the Buddha's Emanation Body.

Similitudes of a Buddha's three bodies can be identified not only for the path, but also for the ordinary states of sleep and death. When one goes to sleep, the mind of clear light is momentarily experienced (though not, ordinarily, remembered later); this mind of clear light of sleep is like the Buddha's Truth Body, which is the mind of actual clear light. After one is asleep, a dream body may arise; this dream body, which is a type of illusory body, is like the Buddha's Complete Enjoyment Body, which is a pure illusory body. Finally, when the dream body re-enters the coarse body, it is like the Buddha's emanation of a body to serve the welfare of sentient beings.

Similarly, at the time of death, one experiences the mind of clear light of death, which is similar to the Buddha's mind of clear light, the Truth Body; when one rises in an illusory body in place of the intermediate state body, one has a body like the Buddha's Complete Enjoyment Body; and when one uses another body or series of bodies to complete the path, it is like the Buddha's Emanation Body.

Also, just in the ordinary state in general, the mind of clear light at the time of death is like the Buddha's Truth

Chart 9. *Correlations to the Bodies of the Buddha*

Body of Buddha	Entity of Body	Correlation to Ordinary States	Correlation to Single Day	Correlation to Path	Correlation to Sleep	Correlation to Death
Truth Body	Actual Clear Light	Clear Light of Death	Deep Sleep	Actual Clear Light	Mind of Clear Light	Mind of Clear Light
Complete Enjoyment Body	Pure Illusory Body	Intermediate State	Dreaming	Impure Illusory Body	Dream Body	Illusory Body in Place of Intermediate State Body
Emanation Body	Emanated Forms	Conception	Waking	Re-enter Coarse Body	Re-enter Coarse Body	Emanation Body Used to Complete Path

5 Clear Light

The definition of the level of clear light is:[191]

the stages of completion ranging from the proximate causes that are methods for manifesting the clear light up to but not including the attainment of union.

The actual clear light is the mind of great bliss that directly realizes emptiness. Simultaneous with its manifestation, all of the obstructions to liberation — the subtle conception of inherent existence and its karmic seeds — are completely destroyed.

Minds of clear light are the fundamental consciousnesses of all beings, ranging from hell-beings to Buddhas. It is the type of mind into which all beings die and out of which all beings are born[192] in the sense that it is always experienced at the moment of death and again at the moment of conception. For most beings, their mind of clear light is experienced only at times when they have no control over it and no cognizance of it — at death, when going to sleep, and so forth. Buddhas, on the other hand, operate only from within it, for Buddhas remain continuously in the mind of clear light, realizing emptiness totally non-dualistically while dualistically realizing all other phenomena with emanations filling the universe for the welfare of others.

The mind of clear light manifests when all of the winds are totally dissolved into the indestructible drop in the heart. The total withdrawal of winds teamed with great bliss makes it an extraordinarily powerful means for realizing the nature of reality, emptiness.

The other three empties — white appearance, red increase, and black near-attainment — leading up to clear light are its proximate or immediately preceding causes*. Those three empties are, except for the mind of clear light itself, the most subtle of all consciousnesses and are the last three minds experienced prior to the mind of actual clear light. Though the definition of the *level* of clear light includes them within the level of clear light, they are not themselves clear lights. Conversely, it is possible for a particular mind of clear light not to be of the *level* of clear light. For example, minds of clear light experienced at the time of death are not actual clear lights because they are not even path consciousnesses. Also, minds of clear light experienced at earlier levels of the stage of completion are "metaphoric" clear lights and not of the level of actual clear light because they are conceptual consciousnesses, tainted by subtle dualism. Furthermore, the mind of clear light of the level of a learner's or non-learner's union is a mind of clear light but is not of the level of clear light.

Attaining Clear Light After Sutra Paths

Although the other three empties are the immediately preceding or proximate causes of the actual clear light, the basic prerequisites for attaining the actual clear light are either the attainment of the impure illusory body or the accumulation of merit over three periods of countless great aeons. In general, tantric Bodhisattvas attain the impure illusory body as a prerequisite for attaining the actual clear light whereas sutra Bodhisattvas accumulate merit for three periods of countless great aeons.

Because Shākyamuni Buddha accumulated merit for three periods of countless great aeons, he was able to actualize the clear light without having to attain the impure illusory body, which would have required the use of a consort. This does not mean, however, that he became enlightened in his coarse body, nor that he shunned the use of a consort on the path. At the end of his last lifetime prior to enlightenment, he attained the last of the ten Bodhisattva grounds (the ten levels of the path of meditation, which immediately precede the path of no more learning, i.e., Buddhahood). He was taken to a Highest Pure Land where in his tantric practice he eventually joined with a consort named Hlay-bu-mo Tik-lay-chok-ma or Devī Tilottamā[193] (*lha'i bu mo thig le mchog ma*, the "Divine Daughter Whose Drop is Supreme"). He received instructions and initiations from previous Buddhas, actualized the clear light, the pure illusory body, and union, whereupon he became completely enlightened; later, he emanated a human body, the historical Shākyamuni, to teach the Doctrine.[194]

There are two slightly different explanations for how the actual clear light can be manifested after sutra paths. The first, by Yang-jen-ga-way-lo-drö, the teacher of Nga-wang-bel-den, is that when one reaches the last of the ten grounds of the Perfection Vehicle (a point at which one has abandoned the afflictive obstructions and a certain portion of the obstructions to omniscience) one dwells in meditative equipoise in a Highest Pure Land until aroused by the fingersnaps and exhortations of all the Buddhas. They bestow on one the third of the four tantric initiations (i.e., the wisdom initiation, which requires a consort) at midnight, and this enables one to manifest the four empties. At dawn, they give one further instructions on the clear light and union — the last initiation (the word initiation) — enabling one to rise in a learner's union, the pure illusory body with the mind of actual clear light. Shortly thereafter, in the third portion of the dawn, one attains a non-learner's union, Buddhahood, the simultaneous union of the pure illusory body and actual clear light devoid even of the obstructions to omniscience.

The other explanation of enlightenment at the end of the

sutra paths is that of Dzong-ka-ba's disciple Kay-drup, who explains that with the third initiation one is also "set up" with further instructions (apparently the fourth initiation). Through the third initiation, one realizes emptiness with great bliss (the mind of actual clear light), and then, through the force of the previous set-up, one rises in a body of union.

Those who attain Buddhahood after the complete traversal of the sutra paths always attain it in a Highest Pure Land, whereas those who practice tantra prior to completing the sutra paths can attain enlightenment within the Desire Realm* itself, and those who practice vajra repetition and withdrawal at the time of death can attain enlightenment in place of the intermediate state.[195]

Types of Clear Light
The term "clear light" can refer either to a subject or an object. The objective clear light* is emptiness; it is the clear light that is to be realized. The subjective clear light* is the mind realizing emptiness and can be sub-divided into subjective clear lights that conceptually realize emptiness and subjective clear lights that directly realize emptiness. The subjective clear light that is the conceptual realization of emptiness is called the metaphoric clear light and the subjective clear light that is the direct realization of emptiness is called the actual clear light. The actual clear light of the fourth stage is also spoken of both as "external manifest enlightenment" because it is always initially manifested at dawn (just as Shākyamuni Buddha became enlightened at dawn) and as "internal manifest enlightenment" because it is the all-empty clear light into which all other minds have dissolved.

There are three other ways on the stage of completion of speaking about clear light, in terms of the "general" meaning, "hidden" meaning, and "final" meaning of clear light (see chart 10). There are two general meanings of clear light; the first is clear light in the sense of a coarse mental consciousness that realizes emptiness. Hence, in this general meaning of clear light, a mind of clear light is experienced even in the Perfection Vehicle (the sutra paths) and the three lower tantras because they also include such minds that realize emptiness. The second general meaning of clear light is in the sense of a "melting" bliss consciousness — one generated due to the melting and dripping of the drops in the channels — that realizes emptiness. This type of consciousness is also not unique to the Highest Yoga Tantra stage of completion, for it can be experienced even on the stage of generation.

The "hidden" meaning of clear light is the metaphoric clear light, the ordinarily hidden subtle consciousness that does not become manifest until winds dissolve in the central channel. The metaphoric clear lights that occur on the levels of physical, verbal, and mental isolation, and impure illusory body are this clear light.

The actual clear light is the final meaning of clear light, the final mode of realizing emptiness by a consciousness of innate bliss. It is final in the sense of being the "final quality" or highest level of mind.[196]

Chart 10. *Meanings of Clear Light*

Type	Meaning	System or Level
General Meaning	(1) Coarse Mental Consciousness that Realizes Emptiness	Perfection Vehicle, All Four Sets of Tantras
	(2) Melting Bliss Consciousness that Realizes Emptiness	Stages of Generation and Completion
Hidden Meaning	Metaphoric Clear Light (Bliss Consciousness that Realizes Emptiness, Due to Withdrawal of Winds in Central Channel)	Physical, Verbal, Mental Isolations, Impure Illusory Body, Union of Abandonment of Learner's Union
Final Meaning	Actual Clear Light (Final Mode of Realizing Suchness by Innate Bliss)	Clear Light, Learner's Union, Non-Learner's Union

6 Learner's Union

The definition of a learner's union is:[197]

> the stages of completion taken from rising in a pure illusory body — in dependence on the winds that serve as the mount of the actual clear light of the fourth stage serving as its substantial cause and the mind of clear light serving as its cooperative condition, this arising being simultaneous with slight movement of the winds from that actual clear light of the fourth stage — up through the actual clear light at the end of learning.

After one has experienced the actual clear light, the winds stir slightly again, and one rises in an illusory body that now, due to the destruction of the obstructions to liberation from cyclic existence, is called a pure illusory body. The substantial cause of the pure illusory body is the very subtle fundamental wind, and the cooperative condition of the pure illusory body is the mind of clear light. However, the mind of clear light is not itself manifest at the time of attaining the pure illusory body.[198] Instead, one "reverses" into the mind of black near-attainment and goes back through the other coarser minds. When one has attained the pure illusory body but does not also have the mind of actual clear light, one has attained a union of abandonment*, whereas when one later re-experiences the mind of actual clear light, one attains a realizational union*. That is, when, having risen in a pure illusory body, one again attains the actual clear light, one achieves a realizational union of the pure illusory body and actual clear light.[199]

With the attainment of a learner's union one has simultaneously attained the second Bodhisattva ground and the fourth of the five paths, the path of meditation. Continuing to meditate on emptiness and also to perform other activities while subsisting in a pure illusory body, one again attains the actual clear light. Within the resulting realizational union of the pure illusory body and the actual clear light, one practices until the obstructions to omniscience have been destroyed and thereby passes on to Buddhahood, the non-learner's union of the Form Body and Truth Body, that is, the pure illusory body and the mind of actual clear light, devoid of all obstructions.

From the illusory body one can emanate as many forms as one wishes (including using one's old, coarse body) to act for the benefit of others, thus quickly amassing vast collections of merit.[200] When the collections of merit and wisdom have been completed, the last obstructions to omniscience are eliminated, and the actual clear light and the pure illusory body become the mind and body of a Buddha.

This final union, that of a non-learner, has seven exalted features:[201]

1 one's Complete Enjoyment Body has the thirty-two major and eighty minor marks of a Buddha;
2 one's Complete Enjoyment Body is embracing a Wisdom Seal;
3 one's mind always remains in a state of great bliss;
4 that bliss is always mixed with cognition of emptiness;
5 one's mind never wavers from great compassion for all sentient beings;

6 the continuum of one's body never ceases; and

7 one's emanations pervade the universe ceaselessly performing activities for the benefit of others.

These are the incomparable qualities of a Buddha Superior.

Bringing Death to the Path

The achievement of Buddhahood through the tantric path also brings to a conclusion the tantric process of mimicking death, intermediate state, and rebirth. The quintessential feature of Highest Yoga Tantra is that the ordinary events of death, the intermediate stage, and rebirth are "brought to the path", i.e., mimicked, and transformed into the three bodies — the Truth Body, the Complete Enjoyment Body, and the Emanation Body — of a Buddha[202] (see chart 11). Death is brought to the path in the stage of generation by visualizing the process of the dissolution of elements, etc., as it occurs at the time of death; it is brought to the path in the stage of completion by the actual dissolution of all of the winds in the indestructible drop at the heart at the end of the level of mental isolation, a process that corresponds, in the ordinary state, to dying. The very subtle mind of clear light that dawns upon the dissolution of winds in the indestructible drop at the heart, rather than becoming the clear light of ordinary death, becomes the metaphoric clear light and then the actual clear light, the omniscient consciousness — the Truth Body — of a Buddha.

The intermediate state is brought to the path in the stage of generation by visualizing that one rises up in the form of a mantra seed syllable or as a hand symbol such as a vajra or lotus, and it is brought to the path in the stage of completion by rising in an illusory body, an event that, in the ordinary state, occurs only as one enters the intermediate state between death and rebirth. The very subtle wind that abides in the indestructible drop and ordinarily becomes manifest only at the time of death does not become the substantial cause of the body of the intermediate state being; rather, it becomes the substantial cause of the impure illusory body and then the pure illusory body, which, at the time of a non-learner's union, is the Complete Enjoyment Body of a Buddha. Death, the dissolution of the aggregates due to the exhaustion of their impelling karma, is destroyed.

Birth is brought to the path in the stage of generation by one's appearance as a deity and it is brought to the path in the stage of completion by taking the old body as an Emanation Body after enlightenment, just as one ordinarily assumes a body at the time of conception in the ordinary state.

Chart 11. *Transformation of the Ordinary State in the Path*

Ordinary State	How Brought to Path by Stage of Generation	How Brought to Path by Stage of Completion	Buddha Body Brought to Path
Death	Meditation on Emptiness Following Pattern of Eight Signs of Death	Dissolution of Winds in Indestructible Drop	Truth Body
Intermediate State	Rising in Form of Seed Syllable or Hand Symbol	Rising in an Illusory Body	Complete Enjoyment Body
Rebirth	Appearing as Deity	Taking Old Body as Emanation	Emanation Body

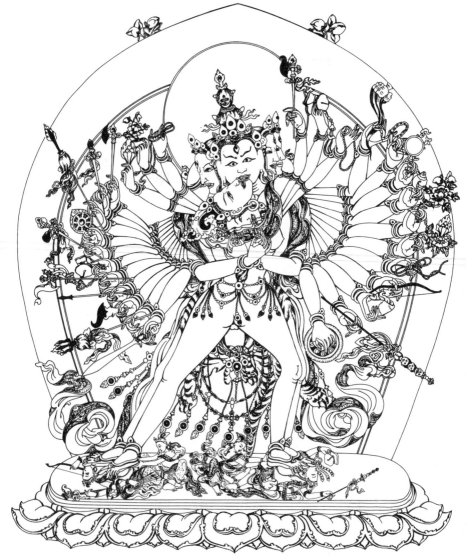

Kālachakra

1 Systems of Highest Yoga Tantra

The Tantric College of Lower Hla-sa teaches eight great tantric systems of instruction for the stage of completion: Nāgārjuna's system of *Guhyasamāja*, Jñānapāda's system of *Guhyasamāja*, Lūhipāda's system of *Chakrasaṃvara*, Ghaṇṭapāda's system of *Chakrasaṃvara*, the system of *Kālachakra*, the system of the three *Yāmaris*, the system of *Mahāchakra*, and the Six Yogas of Nāropa.[203]

With the exception of *Kālachakra*, all of these systems explain similarly the process of achieving complete enlightenment.[204] They say that first one practices the stage of generation and makes it stable (as in the *Guhyasamāja* subtle stage of generation, wherein at the perfection of visualization the entire mandala can be vividly seen in a subtle drop). Then one gains serviceability of the winds and drops through various techniques (such as wind yoga or heat yoga);[205] as a result, winds enter the central channel, bringing about the manifestation of the four empties — the minds of white appearance, red increase, black near-attainment, and clear light. Completing the process of wind-gathering, one rises in an illusory body, subsequently experiences the mind of actual clear light, and finally attains a simultaneous union of the clear light and illusory body. In all of these systems, the actual clear light is the substantial cause of the Buddha's Truth Body, and the illusory body is the substantial cause of his Form Body.

The exception to this scheme is the system of the *Kālachakra Tantra*, which sets forth unique methods for the creation of similitudes of a Buddha's mind and body. Whereas other tantras merely teach methods to separate the very subtle body and mind from the coarse and subtle body and mind, the practice of *Kālachakra* results in the total de-materialization of the coarse body of the elements and their evolutes and the subtle body of drops and winds. The following sections will describe the physiology of the subtle body according to *Kālachakra* and delineate the differences between the *Kālachakra* and *Guhyasamāja* systems with regard to the structure of the tantric paths and the fruits of practice.[207]

2 Channels, Winds, and Drops

The *Kālachakra* system shares with the *Guyhasamāja* system the basic scheme of the channels and winds, with minor differences.[208]

1 In the *Guhyasamāja* system, the right and left channels run parallel to the central channel from top to bottom, but in the *Kālachakra* system, they cross over the central channel at the navel.[209]

2 In the *Guhyasamāja* system, in ordinary waking life the right and left channels contain wind whereas the central channel is absolutely empty. However, according to the *Kālachakra* system, all three channels contain various substances. In the upper part of the body, the right channel contains blood, the left channel contains semen, and the central channel contains wind. In the lower part of the body, the right channel (now on the left due to having crossed-over at the navel) contains feces, the left channel (now on the right) contains urine, and the central channel contains semen.

3 Some of the channel-wheels have a different number of petals, or spokes: in the *Guhyasamāja* system, the crown has thirty-two, the forehead has none, and the throat has sixteen, whereas in the *Kālachakra* system the crown has

four, the forehead has sixteen, and the throat has thirty-two.

4 In *Kālachakra* there are said to be ten winds instead of the five presented in *Guhyasamāja*.[210]

When compared to the other great tantric systems, the most remarkable aspect of the *Kālachakra* scheme is that winds are already moving in the central channel prior to the beginning of tantric practice and before death. It is also remarkable that the lower portion of the central channel is said to contain semen. (In the *Guhyasamāja* system, where the central channel is empty from top to bottom, the pleasure of orgasm is explained by the fact that semen passes *near* the central channel; that is why the presence of the red and white drops *in* the central channel causes a bliss a hundred times greater than that of orgasm.)

The *Kālachakra* system also differs greatly from the *Guhyasamāja* system with regard to the types of drops (see chart 12). As in the *Guhyasamāja* system, there are material red and white drops, but the *Kālachakra* system adds four other types of drops (made from the red and white drops) that normally abide in seven separate locations in the body. The four drops are: (1) body drops, located at the crown and navel, which bear the karmic predispositions involved in wakefulness; (2) speech drops, located at the throat and secret place, which bear the karmic predispositions involved in dreaming; (3) mind drops, located at the heart and center of the sexual organ, which bear the karmic predispositions involved in deep sleep; and (4) exalted wisdom drops, located at the navel and tip of the sexual organ, which bear the karmic predispositions involved in absorption (sexual pleasure). All four types of drops are the size of mustard seeds and are a mixture of red and white drops. The very subtle wind and mind abides in all of them (rather than in an indestructible drop, which is never mentioned), and hence, these drops are the basis for the infusion of karmic predispositions.[211] That being the case, the four drops contain all the obstructions that are to be removed,

```
Gateways Book & Gift
02/13/95    14:08        2019
    1 @   7.25 USED BK       12
SUBTOTAL                 $    7.25
SALES TAX @ 8.25%        $    7.25
TOTAL                    $    0.60
TENDER VISA C            $    7.85
                         $    7.85

1018 Pacific Av S Cruz CA 95060 429-9600
Our TOLL FREE number is (800)459-0055!
```

that is, purified.

The collection of winds at the locations of these drops activates the predispositions infused in them. In wakefulness, many winds gather at the crown of the head and at the navel; in dreaming, many winds gather at the throat and secret place; in deep sleep, many winds gather at the heart and center of the sexual organ; and in sexual union, many winds gather at at the navel and tip of the sexual organ. Due to the activation of karmic predispositions that are located at those places, various pure and impure objects are produced. When one is awake, either pure appearances (such as the body of a deity) or impure appearances are produced; when one is dreaming, either pure "mere sound" (such as mantra) or impure "mistaken speech" are produced; when one is in a dreamless sleep, either pure non-conceptuality (the direct realization of emptiness) or impure unclarity are produced; and when one is in sexual union, either pure bliss (a great bliss consciousness that realizes emptiness) or impure emission of semen are produced. Ordinary persons experience only impure objects, for they are as yet unable to activate the karmic predispositions for the production of pure objects.

The goal of the path is to purify the drops such that only the pure objects — pure appearances, mere sound, non-conceptuality, and bliss — remain, whereas the impure objects — impure appearances, mistaken speech, unclarity, and emission of semen — are precluded. On the path, potencies with the body drops are purified into the "empty forms" (deity bodies devoid of materiality) that will ripen as the Buddha's body, potencies with the speech drops are purified into the mantra sounds that will ripen as the Buddha's speech, and potencies with the mind drops and exalted wisdom drops are purified respectively into the non-conceptual realization of emptiness and the great bliss realizing emptiness that will ripen as the Buddha's mind. In terms of the three bodies of the Buddha, potencies with the body drops become the Emanation Body, potencies with the speech drops become the Complete Enjoyment Body, and potencies with the mind and exalted wisdom drops together become the Truth Body.[212]

In contrast, the *Guhyasamāja* system does not posit body, speech, mind, and exalted wisdom drops, does not say that drops are bases for the infusion of karmic predispositions, and does not have practices aimed at the purification of drops.

Chart 12. *Drops in the **Kālachakra** System*

Type of Drop	Basic Location	Predis-positions	Ordinary Product	Purified Product	Buddha Body
Body Drop	Crown & Navel	Waking	Impure Appear-ances	Pure Appear-ances (Empty Forms)	Emanation Body
Speech Drop	Throat & Secret Place	Dream-ing	Mistaken Speech	Mere Sound (Mantra Sounds)	Complete Enjoyment Body
Mind Drop	Heart & Center of Sexual Organ	Deep Sleep	Unclarity	Non-con-ceptuality (Direct Realization of Emptiness)	Truth Body
Exalted Wisdom Drop	Navel & Tip of Sexual Organ	Sexual Union	Emission of Semen	Bliss (Great Bliss Realizing Emptiness)	Truth Body

3 Levels of the *Kālachakra* Stage of Completion

As in the *Guhyasamāja* system, the *Kālachakra* system[213] seeks to establish the causes for Buddhahood by the generation of a consciousness in which bliss and emptiness are undifferentiably united. In *Kālachakra*, the undifferentiable union of bliss and emptiness refers to supreme immutable bliss and empty form bodies, that is, bodies of the male and female deities which, though they appear as bodies, are devoid of materiality. Still, because both the appearance of empty form bodies in *Kālachakra* and the appearance of oneself as a deity in *Guhyasamāja* are appearances in form of the wisdom that realizes emptiness, and because the "innate" bliss of *Guhyasamāja* is not inferior to the "immutable" bliss of *Kālachakra*,[214] the two systems are not essentially different in their presentation of the union of bliss and realization of emptiness.

The six levels of the *Kālachakra* stage of completion have the same names as the *Guhyasamāja* system's six types of practice according to technique, namely: individual withdrawal, concentration, vitality-stopping, retention, subsequent mindfulness, and meditative stabilization. Despite this, there is little resemblance between the two tantric systems with regard to the actual activities of similarly-named levels.

Chart 13. *Yogas of Levels of* **Kālachakra**

Level	Yoga	Result
Meditative Stabilization	Retention with Great Seal of Empty Form	Dematerialization of Old Body and Production of Empty Form Bodies
Subsequent Mindfulness	Retention with Great Seal of Empty Form	Drops Melt and Flow
Retention	Holding Winds by Vajra Repetition and Pot-Shaped Yoga	Fierce Woman Generated
Vitality-Stopping	Vajra Repetition and Pot-Shaped Yoga	Winds from Right and Left Channels Enter Central Channel
Concentration	Concentration on Drop at Upper Opening of Central Channel	Eleven Day and Night Signs Become Stable
Individual Withdrawal	Concentration on Drop at Upper Opening of Central Channel	Winds Withdraw from Outside and Eleven Day and Night Signs Dawn

(read from bottom up)

Individual Withdrawal

Individual withdrawal, the initial level of the *Kālachakra* stage of completion, is used to collect the winds back from the "doors" of the senses by means of meditative focusing on a drop. This meditation is to be done in complete darkness (it being difficult to restrain the flow of winds through the eye sense-power when there is bright light[215]); thus, in preparation, one has to construct a light-proof cabin in which to conduct one's meditation. The meditation itself is begun at night. Before beginning the meditation session, one binds one's limbs with cloth or rope. Then one rolls one's eyes upwards (closing them halfway), and holds one's observation on the upper opening of the central channel (between the eyebrows), where there is an empty space. What one begins to see there is a tiny blue drop; it contains the predispositions that produce the waking state.[216]

As one gains facility in this meditation, a series of eleven objects appear to the mind, called "night signs" and "day signs".[217] The four night signs are (1) an appearance like smoke, (2) a shimmering appearance like that of a mirage, (3) an appearance like the specks of light given off by fireflies, and (4) an appearance like the sputtering light of a nearly-depleted butter lamp. These four signs are the same mental images that appear to the mind at the time of death during the dissolution of the four elements — earth, water, fire, and wind — of the body, except that the first two signs are reversed in the *Kālachakra* system.[218]

After the night signs dawn, the six day signs[219] arise. They are: the planet *kālāgni* (which is like the sun, or destructive fire, at the end of a great aeon), the sun, the moon, the planet *rāhu* (an eclipse), lightning, and the blue drop itself. The eleventh sign is neither a night or day sign; it is the appearance, in the center of the blue drop, of the outline of Kālachakra and his consort, Vishvamātā, in sexual union. This last sign is a precursor of empty forms (forms devoid of materiality) that, on the fifth level — the level of subsequent mindfulness — will appear in reality.

The eleven signs that dawn in the yoga of individual withdrawal are not those that precede the dawning of the four empties, although they are very similar to the signs accompanying the dissolutions of the elements and winds preceding death or on the stage of completion of *Guhyasa-māja*. They are not signs of the four empties because they are not generated due to the dissolution of winds in the central channel; rather, at the time of individual withdrawal when these signs arise, the winds are merely stopped from going outside from the doors of the senses and have not yet been drawn inside.

Concentration

Concentration is the continuation of the yoga of individual withdrawal (the penetrative focusing on the upper opening of the central channel). It is performed in order to stabilize the eleven night and day signs that arose earlier. When the signs become clear and steady, it indicates that the central channel has been purified, and winds from the right and left channels naturally begin to enter it.[220]

The first two levels of the *Kālachakra* stage of completion merely prepare the central channel for the entry of winds, whereas the two like-named levels in the *Guhyasamāja* system actually cause winds to enter the central channel.

Vitality-Stopping

Vitality-stopping[221] (*prāṇāyāma*) has two phases, (1) vajra repetition, the observation of the "tones" of the breath, and (2) a yoga called "pot-possessing" which puts together the vitalizing and pervasive winds in the central channel. The pot-possessing yoga is the vivid visualization that the winds from the lower part of the body are held in a pot-like configuration below the navel.[222] These practices cause the winds from the right and left channels to flow into the central channel.

Retention

Retention is the holding of the winds inside the central channel. One does this by holding the breath, without exhalation or inhalation, after the winds have been gathered in the central channel by means of vitality-stopping. This causes the Fierce Woman to be generated.

Subsequent Mindfulness

Subsequent Mindfulness involves the use of either an imagined or actual seal (consort) to make the Fierce Woman blaze up, melting the white drop at the top of the head. Also, one performs deeds of any of the three types — elaborative, non-elaborative, or very non-elaborative —

with this seal in order to increase the constituent and keep it from spreading out at the channel wheels.[223] The white drop flows down to the tip of the sexual organ, generating "innate immutable bliss;" it is not emitted, for one has gained control over the winds that ordinarily would cause emission.[224] This drop is the first of 21,600 white drops that descend and pile up in the central channel, forming a white column while 21,600 red drops rise one at a time to the top of the head and pile downwards, forming a parallel red column.[225]

As this process unfolds, one begins to experience the appearances of actual empty form deities; that is, one oneself appears as a deity devoid of materiality. (These appearances, however, are not fully qualified until the end of the next level, meditative stabilization; they gradually become manifest as the drops pile up.[226]) That is because, as each drop piles up or down without any emission, one portion of the material (form) aggregate and karmic winds are consumed and one "immutable bliss" is experienced. The materiality of the *entire* body gradually diminishes because each of the 21,600 portions of the form aggregate pervades the whole body.[227] The ordinary body does not actually *become* an empty form body; rather, it is explained that just as in alchemy, where iron is not transmuted into gold but rather disappears in the presence of the alchemical substance, allowing gold to *appear*, the ordinary body is dematerialized so that an empty form body can appear.[228]

Meditative Stabilization

Meditative stabilization is the continuation of subsequent mindfulness, with perhaps one difference. During subsequent mindfulness, it is said to be sufficient to use any of the three seals (the imaginary Wisdom Seal, actual Action Seal, or Great Seal of Empty Form). Meditative stabilization specifically involves the use of a Great Seal of Empty Form, which is needed to accomplish the complete consumption of the material aggregates.

The perfection of this practice is sufficient to bring about Buddhahood. Gradually, the white and red drops are built up and down, the material aggregates are consumed, the karmic winds are consumed, and one is suffused with supreme immutable bliss. (The drops, it should be noted, also lose their materiality as they pile up and down.) This bliss serves to vastly empower the wisdom consciousness that realizes emptiness, making it possible to quickly overcome the obstructions to liberation and the obstructions to omniscience. At the end of this level, one has completely abandoned all obstructions to Buddhahood and is endowed with both a Buddha's mirror-like wisdom and his body of empty form, which is said to be "like a rainbow".

Chart 14. *Achievement of a Buddha's Body, Speech, and Mind*

Levels of Stage of Completion	Function	Aspect of Buddhahood Achieved
Meditative Stabilization	Entity of Immutable Bliss	Vajra Mind
Subsequent Mindfulness	Proximate Cause of Immutable Bliss	Vajra Mind
Retention	Making Winds Remain in Central Channel, Igniting Fierce Woman	Vajra Speech
Vitality-Stopping	Control of Winds that are Root of Speech (causing winds of right and left channels to enter central channel)	Vajra Speech
Concentration	Make Empty Forms Stable/Purify Central Channel	Vajra Body
Individual Withdrawal	Achieve Empty Forms/Purify Central Channel	Vajra Body

(read from bottom to top)

3 Summary of Differences with Respect to Practice

It is now evident that in several respects there are considerable differences between the *Guhyasamāja* and *Kālachakra* systems of the stage of completion.

(1) With respect to the stages of the path, the first level of the *Guhyasamāja* stage of completion — physical isolation — would not occur in the *Kālachakra* system until the level of vitality-stopping, because it is not until then that winds actually enter the central channel. The first two levels of *Kālachakra* practice would not even be included in the *Guhyasamāja* stage of completion, but would be consigned to the stage of generation. Also, heat yoga (the generation of the Fierce Woman) does not begin in the *Kālachakra* system until the fourth level — retention — whereas in the *Guhyasamāja* system, the Fierce Woman is generated at the first level — physical isolation — and at every subsequent level of the path. Furthermore, in the *Guhyasamāja* system, it is necessary to cause all of the winds to dissolve in the indestructible drop at the heart in the central channel, and for that, it is necessary to generate the Fierce Woman, inner heat, by way of sexual union with an Action Seal. However, in the *Kālachakra* system, the winds are not said to dissolve

into the indestructible drop.

The absence of the Fierce Woman until the fourth level of the *Kālachakra* stage of completion presumably means that there is no experience of the four joys of ascent and descent of the white and red drops until the fifth stage (although, in fact, the four joys are never mentioned; only "supreme immutable bliss" is mentioned as the aspect of bliss).

(2) There are ten signs of the dissolution of the coarse into the subtle instead of the eight posited by the *Guhyasamāja* system, and the order of the first two signs, the appearance of smoke and mirage, is reversed.

(3) The *Kālachakra* system requires the use of a different type of seal — the Great Seal of Empty Form — because it is said that otherwise the drops would not be able to pile up without spreading out at the channel-wheels.

(4) The effect of the piling up of drops is to de-materialize the body, which means that there is no way that the old body could be used as an emanation body as in the *Guhyasamāja* system. (However, if one wished, one could emanate a body like the old one.)

(5) From the point of view of the *Guhyasamāja* system, there would be no way to achieve enlightenment in place of the intermediate state in the *Kālachakra* system because there is no metaphoric clear light or illusory body. According to *Guhyasamāja*, the attainment of the metaphoric clear light is a necessary precondition for attaining enlightenment in the intermediate state; also, if one were to be enlightened in the intermediate state, it would be in an illusory body which takes the place of an intermediate state body. However, the *Kālachakra* system speaks of dematerialization of the form aggregate rather than the manifestation of an illusory body. Since *Kālachakra* practice aims at the dematerialization of the coarse and subtle body in order to destroy the karmic seeds and predispositions preventing liberation and omniscience, it must occur in a coarse body, not in a subtle body such as an intermediate state body.[229]

This means that one could not attempt to become enlightened in the intermediate state as one was dying, contrary to other systems both of tantra and sutra.[230]

(6) In the *Kālachakra* system, unlike the *Guhyasamāja* system, one can generate an empty form — an appearance of the fundamental mind — without actualizing the fundamental mind itself.

(7) Finally, whereas in *Guhyasamāja* the fundamental wind is the substantial cause of the pure illusory body, in *Kālachakra* there is no mention of any substantial cause of the empty form body.[231]

4 The Five Paths and Ten Grounds

The paths leading to enlightenment in the sutra system are five: accumulation, preparation, seeing, meditation, and no more learning. A practitioner of the Great Vehicle reaches the path of accumulation upon making a firm determination to attain highest enlightenment with the altruistic motivation of being the greatest source of help to others. The path of preparation is attained through conceptual realization of emptiness by a consciousness that is a union of special insight and calm abiding. The path of seeing and the first bodhisattva ground is reached by the direct realization of emptiness. Subsequently, the realization of emptiness is deepened and enhanced by meditation and the practice of the perfections on the path of meditation (which is composed of the remaining nine bodhisattva grounds), culminating in Buddhahood, the path of no more learning.

When the *Guhyasamāja* and *Kālachakra* stages of completion are correlated to the five paths and ten grounds, it is clear that the breakdown of *Kālachakra* levels is weighted more to the paths of accumulation and preparation than is the system of *Guhyasamāja*. Five of the six *Kālachakra* levels are correlated to the paths of accumulation and preparation, whereas only the first three *Guhyasamāja* levels —

physical, verbal, and mental isolation — are equivalent to those sutra paths.

In the *Guhyasamāja* stage of completion, one passes from the path of accumulation (which begins with the generation of the altruistic aspiration to enlightenment by way of the *Guhyasamāja* system) to the path of preparation when winds begin to enter and dissolve in the central channel; this occurs at the very beginning of the stage of completion when the subtle stage of generation becomes the level of physical isolation of the stage of completion. One remains on the path of preparation through the level of impure illusory body, passing to the path of seeing at the first moment of manifesting the mind of actual clear light. The path of meditation is coextensive with the level of learner's union. It can be divided into nine bodhisattva grounds according to the enhancement of the bliss consciousness that realizes emptiness, the increase in the number of one's exalted qualities, and so forth.[232] The path of no more learning, the path of a Buddha, is the non-learner's union.

In the *Kālachakra* system, on the other hand, the path of preparation does not begin until the first white drop reaches the tip of the sexual organ on the fifth level, the level of subsequent mindfulness. The path of seeing (the first direct realization of emptiness) occurs when the white drops have piled up to a point halfway to the secret place, that is, at the 1,800th drop, at the beginning of the level of meditative stabilization.[233] There are twelve bodhisattva grounds in the *Kālachakra* system as opposed to the ten grounds in the sutra and *Guhyasamāja* layouts,[234] and the other eleven grounds are attained in the same way: one passes from one ground to the next with the completion of each series of 1800 drops. This reflects the fact that with the descent of each successive drop, the ignition of bliss becomes more intense, enhancing the realization of emptiness. The level of meditative stabilization develops right into Buddhahood, the path of no more learning.

Glossary
Bibliography
Notes
Index

Glossary

(Asterisk denotes reconstruction of Sanskrit)

English	Sanskrit	Tibetan
achievement	pratipad	sgrub pa
action	karma	las
Action Seal	karmamudrā	las rgya
Action Tantra	kriyātantra	bya rgyud
actual clear light		don gyi 'od gsal
aeon	kalpa	bskal pa
afflictive obstructions/ obstructions to liberation	kleśāvaraṇa	nyon mong pa'i sgrib pa
aggregate	skandha	phung po
altruistic aspiration to enlightenment	bodhicitta	byang chub kyi sems
analysis	vicāra	dpyod pa
appearance	pratibhāsa	snang ba
attachment	tṛṣṇā	sred pa/'dod chags
basic winds		rtsa ba'i rlung
beginner	ādikarmika	las dang po pà
bliss	sukha	bde ba
Bodhisattva	bodhisattva	byang chub sems dpa'

English	*Sanskrit*	*Tibetan*
body	kāya	lus/sku
branch	aṅga	yan lag
Buddha	buddha	sangs rgyas
calm abiding	śamatha	zhi gnas
cause	hetu	rgyu
central channel	avadhūtī	rtsa dbu ma
channel	nāḍī	rtsa
channel-knot		rtsa mdud
channel-wheel	cakra	rtsa 'khor
clear light	prabhāsvara	'od gsal
coarse	audārika	rags pa
Complete Enjoyment Body	sambhogakāya	longs sku
collection	saṃbhāra	tshogs
compassion	karuṇā	snying rje
concentration	dhyāna	bsam gtan
conceptuality	vikalpa/kalpanā	rnam rtog/rtog pa
consciousness	jñā/vijñāna	shes pa/rnam shes
Consequence School	prāsaṅgika	thal 'gyur pa
continuum	saṃtāna	rgyun/rgyud
conventional mind of enlightenment	saṃvṛtibodhicitta	kun rdzob byang chub kyi sems
conventional truth	saṃvṛtisatya	kun rdzob bden pa
correct view	samyakdṛṣṭi	yang dag pa'i lta ba
cyclic existence	saṃsāra	'khor ba
deeds	caryā	spyod pa
deity	deva	lha
deity yoga	devayoga	lha'i rnal 'byor
desire	rāga	'dod chags
Desire Realm	kāmadhātu	'dod khams
direct cognition		mngon sum du rtogs pa
divine pride	devamana	lha'i nga rgyal
Doctrine	dharma	chos

English	Sanskrit	Tibetan
downward-voiding wind		thur sel gyi rlung
drops	bindu	thig le
effort	vīrya	brtson 'grus
eighty indicative conceptions		rang bzhin brgyad cu'i kun rtog
elaborations	prapañca	spros pa
Emanation Body	nirmāṇakāya	sprul sku
empowerment/ initiation	abhiśeka	dbang
emptiness	śūnyatā	stong ba nyid
empty	śūnya	stong pa
enlightenment	bodhi	byang chub
ethics	śīla	tshul khrims
exalted wisdom of emptiness		stong pa'i ye shes
excitement	auddhatya	rgod pa
exertion	vyāyāma	rtsol ba
Fierce Woman	caṇḍālī	gtum mo
fire-dwelling wind		mnyam gnas kyi rlung
Foe Destroyer	arhan/arhat	dgra bcom pa
form/visible form	rūpa	gzugs
Form Body	rūpakāya	gzugs sku
Form Realm	rūpadhātu	gzugs khams
giving	dāna	sbyin pa
great aeon	mahākalpa	bskal pa chen po
Great Vehicle	mahāyāna	theg chen
ground	bhūmi	sa
Highest Pure Land	akaniṣṭha	'og min
Highest Yoga Tantra	anuttarayogatantra	rnal 'byor bla med kyi rgyud
ignorance	avidyā	ma rig pa
illusory body	māyādeha	sgyu lus

English	Sanskrit	Tibetan
imprint		lag rjes
increase	vrddhiprāpta	mched pa
inestimable mansion	*amātragrha/ *sumātragrha	gzhal med khang/gzhal yas khang
inhalation	āna/śvāsa	dbugs rngub pa
inherent establishment	svabhāvasiddha	rang bzhin gyis grub pa
initial joining		dang po sbyor ba
initiation/ empowerment	abhiśeka	dbang
innate joy	sahajānanda	lhan rkyes kyi dga' ba
intermediate state	antarābhāva	bar do
isolation	viveka	dben
joy	ānanda	dga' ba
Knowledge Woman	vidyā	rig ma
knowledge-wisdom initiation	prajñājñānābhiśeka	shes rab ye shes kyi dbang
lama	guru	bla ma
latencies/ predispositions	vāsanā	bag chags
laxity	laya	bying ba
learner	śiṣya	slob pa
left channel	lalanā	brkyang ma
liberation	mokṣa	thar pa
light drop	ābhāsabindu	'od thig
mandala	maṇḍala	dkhyil 'khor
manifest	abhimukhî	mngon gyur
mantra	mantra	snags
mantra drop	mantrabindu	snags thig
means of achievement	sādhana	sgrub thabs

English	Sanskrit	Tibetan
meditative equipoise	samāhita	mnyam bzhag
meditative stabilization	samādhi	ting nge 'dzin
mental continuum	cittasaṃtāna	sems rgyud
mental isolation		sems dben
merit	puṇya	bsod nams
metaphoric clear light		dpe'i 'od gsal
method	upāya	thabs
Middle Way School	mādhyamika	dbu ma pa
middling	madhya	'bring
mind	citta	sems
mind of enlightenment/altruistic aspiration to enlightenment	bodhicitta	byang chub kyi sems
Mind-Only School	cittamātra	sems tsam pa
mindfulness	smṛti	dran pa
motivation		kun slong
Nature Truth Body	svabhāvikakāya	ngo bo nyid sku
near-attainment	ālokasyopalabdhiśa	nyer thob
non-conceptual	nirvikalpaka	rtog med
obstructions to liberation/afflictive obstructions	kleśāvaraṇa	nyon mongs pa'i sgrib pa
obstructions to omniscience	jñeyāvaraṇa	shes bya'i sgrib pa
path	mārga	lam
path of accumulation	saṃbhāramārga	tshogs lam
path of meditation	bhāvanāmārga	sgom lam
path of no more learning	aśaikṣamārga	mi slob lam

English	Sanskrit	Tibetan
path of preparation	prayogamārga	sbyor lam
path of seeing	darśanamārga	mthong lam
patience	kṣānti	bzod pa
Perfection of Wisdom	prajñāpāramitā	shes rab kyi phar rol tu phyin pa
Perfection Vehicle	pāramitāyāna	phar phyin theg pa
Performance Tantra	caryātantra	spyod rgyud
pervasive wind		khyab byed kyi rlung
phenomenon	dharma	chos
physical isolation		lus dben
pledge	samaya	dam tshig
pledge-being	samayasattva	dam tshig pa
pot-possessing yoga		bum pa can gyi rnal 'byor
predisposition/ latency	vāsanā	bag chags
pride	māna	nga rgyal
Pure Land	kṣetraśuddhi	dag zhing
realization		rtogs pa
realizational union		rtogs pa zung 'jug
renunciation	niḥsaraṇa	nges 'byung
[restraining] vitality and exertion	prāṇāyāma	srog rtsol
retention	dhāraṇa	'dzin pa
right channel	rasanā	rtsa ro ma
seal	mudrā	phyag rgya
secondary winds		yan lag gi rlung
secret empowerment	guhyābhiṣeka	gsang dbang
Secret Mantra Vehicle	guhyamantrayāna	gsang sngags kyi theg pa
sense power	indriya	dbang po
sentient being	sattva	sems can
similar in aspect	*ākārabhāgīya	rnam pa dang mthun pa

English	Sanskrit	Tibetan
special insight	vipaśyanā	lhag mthong
special joy	virmānanda	khyad par gyi dga' ba
Spiritual Community	saṃgha	dge 'dun
stability		gnas cha
stage of completion	niṣpannakrama	rdzogs rim
stage of generation	utpattikrama	bskyed rim
subsequent mindfulness	anusmṛti	rjes dran
substance drop	dravyabindu	rdzas thig
subtle		phra ba
Superior	ārya	'phags pa
supreme joy	paramānanda	mchog dga'
supreme king of actions		las rgyal mchog
supreme king of mandalas		dkyil 'khor rgyal mchog
sutra	sūtra	mdo
tantra	tantra	rgyud
tenet system	siddhānta	grub mtha'
those upon whom a little wisdom has descended		ye shes cung zad babs pa
those who have achieved slight mastery with respect to wisdom		ye shes la cung zad dbang thob pa
those who have achieved thorough mastery with respect to wisdom		ye shes la yang dag par dbang thob pa
Truth Body	dharmakāya	chos sku

English	Sanskrit	Tibetan
ultimate mind of enlightenment	paramārtha-bodhicitta	don dam byang chub kyi sems
ultimate truth	paramārthasatya	don dam bden pa
union	yuganaddha	zung 'jug
union of abandonment		spangs pa zung 'jug
upward-moving wind		gyen rgyu'i rlung
vagina	bhaga	bha ga
vajra repetition	vajrajāpa	rdo rje bzlas pa
vase initiation		bum dbang
vehicle	yāna	theg pa
vitality-lengthening		srog sing
vitalizing wind		srog 'dzin kyi rlung
vow	saṃvara	sdom pa
wind (element)	vāyu	rlung
wind (vital energy)	prāṇa	rlung
wind yoga	prāṇāyāma	srog rtsol
wisdom	prajñā	shes rab
wisdom being	jñānasattva	ye shes pa
Wisdom Seal	jñānamudrā	ye shes kyi phyag rgya
Wisdom Truth Body	jñānadharmakāya	ye shes chos sku
withdrawal	pratyāhāra	sor 'dus
word initiation		tshig dbang
wrong consciousness	mithyājñāna	log shes
yoga	yoga	rnal 'byor
yoga of single-mindedness of the coarse		rags pa dran pa gcig pa'i rnal 'byor
yoga realizing the subtle		phra ba rtog pa'i rnal 'byor
Yoga Tantra	yogatantra	rnal 'byor rgyud

Bibliography

Note: "P" refers to the Peking edition of the *Tibetan Tripitaka* (Tokyo-Kyoto: Tibetan Tripitaka Research Foundation, 1956).

1. Selected Tantras

Guhyasamāja Tantra
    sarvatathāgatakāyavākcittarahasyaguhyasamājanāmamahākal-
        parāja/de bzhin gshegs pa thams cad kyi sku gsung thugs kyi
        gsang chen gsang ba 'dus pa zhes bya ba brtag pa'i rgyal po
        chen po
    P 81, Vol. 3
Kālachakra Tantra
    paramādibuddhoddhṛtaśrīkālacakranāmatantrarāja/ mchog gi
        dang po'i sang rgyas las byung ba rgyud kyi rgyal po dpal dus
        kyi 'khor lo
    P 4, Vol. 1

2. Sanskrit and Tibetan Texts Cited in This Book

Chandrakīrti (zla ba grags pa, 7th century)

146 Bibliography

Brilliant Lamp, Extensive Commentary [on the "Guhyasamāja Tantra"]
pradīpoddyotananamatika/sgron ma gsal bar byed pa zhes bya ba'i rgya cher bshad pa
P 2650, Vol. 60.

Commentary on (Nāgārjuna's) "Sixty Stanzas of Reasoning"
yuktiṣaṣṭikāvṛtti/rigs pa drug cu pa'i grel pa
P 5265, Vol. 98.

Dzong-ka-ba (tsong kha pa blo bzang grags pa, 1357-1419)

Lamp Thoroughly Illuminating (Nāgārjuna's) "The Five Stages": Quintessential Instructions of the King of Tantras, The Glorious Guhyasamāja
rgyud kyi rgyal po dpal gsang ba 'dus pa'i man ngag rim pa lnga rab tu gsal ba'i sgron me
P 6167, Vol. 158. Also: Varanasi, 1969.

Great Exposition of Secret Mantra
rgyal ba khyab bdag rdo rje 'chang chen po'i lam gyi rim pa gsang ba kun gyi gnad rnam par phye ba, also known as sngags rim chen mo
Dharmsala: Shes rig par khang, 1969. Also: *Collected Works*, Vol. 4 (New Delhi: Ngawang Gelek Demo, 1975).
Sections on Action and Performance Tantras translated by Jeffrey Hopkins as *Tantra in Tibet: The Great Exposition of Secret Mantra.* (London: George Allen & Unwin, 1977) and *Yoga of Tibet: The Great Exposition of Secret Mantra, Parts 2 and 3* (London: George Allen & Unwin, 1981).

Middling Exposition of the Stages of the Path
lam rim chung ba (lam rim 'bring)
P 6002, Vol. 132. Also: Dharmsala: Shes rig par khang, 1968.
Translation of section on special insight by Jeffrey Hopkins (unpublished); also, Robert A. F. Thurman, *Life and Teaching of Tsong Khapa*, (Dharmsala: Library of Tibetan Works and Archives, 1983).

Precious Sprout, a Final Analysis
mtha' gcod rin po che'i myu gu/ rgyud kyi rgyal po dpal gsang ba 'dus pa'i rgya cher bshad pa sgron ma gsal ba'i dka' ba'i gnas kyi mtha' gcod
P 6152, Vol. 156.

Three Principal Aspects of the Path

lam gyi gtso bo rnam pa gsum

P 6087, Vol. 153.

Translated by Geshe Wangyal, *The Door of Liberation*, pp. 128-30, and Robert A. F. Thurman, *Life and Teachings of Tsong Khapa*, pp. 57-8.

Jam-yang-shay-ba ('jam dbyangs bzhad pa, 1648-1721)

Great Exposition of Tenets/ Explanation of "Tenets", Sun of the Land of Samantabhadra Brilliantly Illuminating All of Our Own and Others' Tenets and the Meaning of the Profound, Ocean of Scripture and Reasoning Fulfilling All Hopes of All Beings

grub mtha'i rnam bshad rang gzhan grub mtha' kun dang zab don mchog tu gsal ba kun bzang zhing gi nyi ma lung rigs rgya mtsho skye dgu'i re ba kun skong

Mussorie: Dalama, 1962.

Presentation of the Seventy Topics

dngos po brgyad don bdun cu'i rnam bzhag legs par bshad pa'i mi pham blo ma'i zhal lung

Volume 15 of *Collected Works* (Delhi: Ngawang Gelek Demo, 1973).

Jang-gya Rol-bay-dor-jay (lcang skya rol pa'i rdo rje, 1717-86)

Presentation of Tenets/Clear Exposition of the Presentations of Tenets, Beautiful Ornament for the Meru of the Subduer's Teaching

grub mtha'i rnam bzhag/grub pa'i mtha'i rnam par bzhag pa gsal bar bshad pa thub bstan lhun po'i mdzes rgyan

Varanasi: Pleasure of Elegant Sayings Press, 1970. Also: *Collected Works* (New Delhi: Mongolian Lama Guru Deva, 1982).

Kay-drup-ge-lek-bel-sang (mkhas grub dge legs dpal bzang, 1385-1438)

Ocean of Feats, the Stage of Generation

bskyed rim dngos grub rgya mtsho/rgyud thams cad kyi rgyal po dpal gsang ba 'dus pa'i bskyed rim dngos grub rgya mtsho

Toh. 5481, Vol. 59.

Lo-sang-gyel-tsen-seng-gay (blo bzang rgyal mtshan seng ge, born 1757/8)

Presentation of the Stage of Completion of the Lone Hero, The Glorious Vajrabhairava, Cloud of Offerings Pleasing Mañjushri

dpal rdo rje 'jigs byed dpa' bo gcig pa'i rdzogs rim gyi rnam bzhag 'jam dpal dgyes pa'i mchod sprin
Delhi: 1972.

Nga-wang-bel-den (ngag dbyang dpal ldan, b. 1797)

Illumination of the Texts of Tantra, Presentation of the Grounds and Paths of the Four Great Secret Tantra Sets
gsang chen rgyud sde bzhi'i sa lam gyi rnam bzhag gzhung gsal byed
rgyud smad par khang edition, no other data. This is the edition used for this book. Also: *The Collected Works of Chos-rje Nag-dbaṅ-dpal-ldan of Urga*, Volume II (Delhi: Mongolian Lama Guru Deva, 1983).

Paṇ-chen Sö-nam-drak-ba (pan chen bsod nams grags pa, 1478-1554)

General Presentation of the Tantra Sets, Captivating the Minds of the Fortunate
rgyud sde spyi'i rnam par bzhag pa skal bzang gi yid 'phrog
Dharmsala: Library of Tibetan Works and Archives, 1975.

Shāntideva (zhi ba lha)

Engaging in the Bodhisattva Deeds
bodhisattvacaryāvatāra/byang chub sems dpa'i spyod pa la 'jug pa
P 5272, Vol. 99.

Sanskrit and Tibetan texts: *Bodhicaryāvatāra of Sāntideva*, ed. by Vidhushekhara Bhattacharya (Calcutta: Asiatic Society, 1960).

Translated by Stephen Batchelor as *Guide to the Bodhisattva's Way of Life* (Dharmsala: Library of Tibetan Works and Archives, 1979).

Yang-jen-ga-way-lo-drö (dbyangs can dga ba'i blo gros, also known as A-gya Yong-dzin [a kya yongs 'dzin], eighteenth century)

Lamp Thoroughly Illuminating the Presentation of the Three Basic Bodies — Death, Intermediate State, and Rebirth
gzhi'i sku gsum gyi rnam gzhag rab gsal sgron me
The Collected Works of A-kya Yongs-'dzin, Vol. 1 (New Delhi: Lama Guru Deva, 1971).

Translated and introduced by Lati Rinbochay and Jeffrey Hopkins as *Death, Intermediate State, and Rebirth in Tibetan Buddhism.* (Ithaca, N.Y.: Snow Lion Publications,

1979).

Presentation of the Grounds and Paths of Mantra According to the Superior Nāgārjuna's Interpretation of the Glorious Guhyasa-māja, A Good Explanation Serving as a Port for the Fortunate. dpal gsang ba 'dus 'pa phags lugs dang mthun pa'i snags kyi sa lam rnam gzhag legs bshad skal bzang 'jug ngogs rnam rgyal grwa tsang, 1969.

3. Other Works

Bagchi, Prabodh Chandra. Studies in the Tantras. Calcutta (n.p.), 1939.

Beyer, Stephen. The Cult of Tara. Berkeley: University of California Press, 1973.

———. The Buddhist Experience: Sources and Interpretations. Encino, Calif.: Dickenson Pub., 1974.

Bharati, Agehananda. The Tantric Tradition. New York: Samuel Weiser, 1975.

———. "Śakta and Vajrayāna: Their Place in Indian Thought," in Studies of Esoteric Buddhism and Tantrism. Koya San: Koya San University, 1965, pp. 73-79.

———. "Intentional Language in the Tantras," Journal of the American Oriental Society 81 (1961), pp. 261-270.

Bhattacharya, Benoytosh. An Introduction to Buddhist Esoterism. London: Oxford University Press, 1932; 2nd ed., 1964

———. "Tantric Cults Among the Buddhists," in Cultural heritage of India, ed. H. D. Bhattacharya, vol. II, pp. 208-21. Calcutta: Ramakrishna Mission Institute of Culture, 1950-60.

———. Guhyasamāja or Tathāgataguhyaka. (ed.) Gaekwad's Oriental Series #53. Baroda: Oriental Institute, 1931.

———. Sādhanamāla. (ed.) Gaekwad's Oriental Series #41. Baroda; Oriental Institute, 1928.

———. Buddhist Iconography. Calcutta: Fa. K. L. Mukhopadhyay, 1959 (reprint of 1924 London edition).

Bhattacharyya, Narendra Nath. History of Researches on Buddhism. New Delhi: Munishram Manoharlal, 1981, pp. 86-99.

Blofeld, John. The Way of Power. London: George Allen & Unwin, 1970.

Bolles, Kee W. "Devotion and Tantra," in Studies of Esoteric

Buddhism and Tantrism. Koya San: Koya San University, 1965, pp. 217-228.

Bromage, Bernard. *Tibetan Yoga.* New York: Samuel Weiser, 1952.

Chandra, Lokesh. *Materials for a History of Tibetan Literature.* Delhi: International Academy of Indian Culture, 1963.

Chang, Garma C.C. *The Six Yogas of Naropa & Teachings on Mahamudra.* Ithaca, N.Y.: Snow Lion Publications, 1986 (2nd ed.), (Orig. pub. as *Teachings of Tibetan Yoga,* 1963).

Ch'en, Kenneth. "Transformations in Buddhism in Tibet," *Philosophy East and West* 7 (Jan. 1958), pp. 117-126.

Conze, Edward. *Buddhism: Its Essence and Development.* New York: Philosophical Library, 1951.

———. *Buddhist Texts Through the Ages.* New York: Harper & Row, 1964.

Dasgupta, N. Y. "Doctrinal Changes — Tantrik Buddhism, Vajrayāna, Kālachakrayāna, Sahajayāna," in *The Struggle for Empire,* Vol. V of *The History and Culture of the Indian People,* ed. K. L. M. Munshi. Bombay: Bharatiya Vidya Bhavan, 1959.

Dasgupta, Sh. B. *An Introduction to Tantric Buddhism.* Berkeley: Shambala Press, 1974.

———. *Obscure Religious Cults.* Calcutta: Firma K. L. Mukhopadhyay, 1962 (second ed.).

Dawa-samdup, Lama Kazi (ed. and trans.) *Śrīcakrasaṃbharatantra* in *Tantric Texts,* VII and XI (ed. Arthur Avalon). Delhi: Motilal Banarsidass, 1977 (reprint of 1913 ed.).

Dutt, Nalinaksha. "Tantric Buddhism," *Bulletin of Tibetology* 1, no. 2 (Oct. 1964), pp. 5-16.

Drub, Gendun, Dalai Lama I. *Selected Works of the Dalai Lama I: Bridging the Sutras and Tantras* (Glenn H. Mullin, trans.). Ithaca; N.Y.: Snow Lion Publications, 1985.

Elder, George. "Problems of Language in Buddhist Tantra," *History of Religions* 15 (Feb. 1976), pp. 231-250.

Eliade, Mircea. *Patañjali and Yoga.* New York: Schocken Books, 1975, 1976.

———. *The Sacred and the Profane.* New York: Harper & Row, 1961.

———. *Yoga: Immortality and Freedom.* New York: Pantheon, 1958.

Evans-Wentz, W. (ed.). *Tibetan Yoga and Secret Doctrines*, trans. Lama Kazi Dawa-Samdup. Oxford University Press, 1928.

Filliozat-Jean "Le complexe d'oedipe dans un tantra Bouddhique," in Bareau (ed.), *Etudes Tibetaines* Paris: Librairie D'Amerique et d'Orient, 1971.

Finot, Louis. "Manuscrits sanskrits de Sādhanas retrouves en Chine," *Journal Asiatique*, 225 (1934).

Frame, James N. "The Nervous System of the Tantras," *Journal of the West Virginia Philosophical Society* 12 (Spring 1977) pp. 20-23.

Getty, Alice. *The Gods of Northern Buddhism*. Rutland, Vermont: Charles E. Tuttle.

George, Christopher (trans.). *The Caṇḍamahāroṣaṇa Tantra*. New Haven: American Oriental Society, 1974.

Govinda, Lama Anagarika. *Creative Meditation and Multi-Dimensional Consciousness*. Wheaton, Ill.: Theosophical Publishing House, 1976.

――――. *Foundations of Tibetan Mysticism*. London: Rider and Co., 1959.

――――. "Principles of Buddhist Tantrism," *Bulletin of Tibetology* Vol. 2, No. 1 (1965), pp. 9-16.

――――. "Principles of Tantric Buddhism," in *2500 Years of Buddhism*. New Delhi: Publications Division, Government of India, 1956, pp. 94-104.

Gray, Terrence James Stannus. *Why Lazarus Laughed: The Essential Doctrine, Zen-Advaita-Tantra*. London; Routledge & Kegan Paul, 1960.

Guenther, Herbert V. *Buddhist Philosophy in Theory and Practice*. New York: Penguin Books, 1971.

――――. *The Life and Teaching of Nāropa*. Oxford: Clarendon Press, 1963.

――――. *Matrix of Mystery*. Berkeley: Shambala Publications, 1984.

――――. *Treasures on the Tibetan Middle Way*. Berkeley: Shambala, 1976 (2nd ed.). (orig. pub. as *Tibetan Buddhism Without Mystification*, 1969).

――――. *Yuganaddha — The Tantric View of Life*. Varanasi: Chowkhamba Sanskrit Series, 2nd ed., 1964.

Guenther, Herbert V., and Trungpa, Chogyam. *The Dawn of Tantra*. Berkeley: Shambala Publications, 1975.

Guhyasamāja or Tathāgataguhyaka. (ed. Benoytosh Bhattacharya). Gaekwad's Oriental Series #53. Baroda: Oriental Institute, 1931.

Gyatso, Geshe Kelsang. *The Clear Light of Bliss.* London: Wisdom Publications, 1982.

―――. *Buddhism in the Tibetan Tradition.* London: Routledge & Kegan Paul, 1984.

Gyatso, Tenzin (bstan 'dzin rgya mtsho, Dalai Lama XIV, 1935-). *Kindness, Clarity, and Insight.* Ithaca, N.Y.: Snow Lion Publications, 1984.

―――. *The Kālachakra Tantra: Rite of Initiation.* London: Wisdom Publications, 1985.

Hadano, Hakuyu. "Human Existence in Tantric Buddhism," *Tohoku Daigaku Bungaku Kenkyu-mempo* No. 9, 1958 (*Annual Report of the Faculty of Arts and Letters*, Tohoku University, Sendai).

Hoffmann, H. *The Religions of Tibet.* London: Allen & Unwin, 1961.

Hopkins, Jeffrey. *Meditation on Emptiness.* London: Wisdom Publications, 1983.

―――. *The Tantric Distinction.* London: Wisdom Publications, 1984.

―――. "Reason as the Prime Principle in Tsong kha pa's Delineation of Deity Yoga as the Demarcation Between Sutra and Tantra", *Journal of the International Association of Buddhist Studies*, Vol. 7, No. 2 (1984), pp. 95-115.

Hopkins, Jeffrey (trans. and ed.). *Compassion in Tibetan Buddhism.* Ithaca, N.Y.: Snow Lion Publications, 1980.

―――. *Tantra in Tibet: The Great Exposition of Secret Mantra.* London: George Allen & Unwin, 1977.

―――. *The Yoga of Tibet: The Great Exposition of Secret Mantra, Parts 2 and 3.* London: George Allen & Unwin, 1981.

―――. *The Kālachakra Tantra: Rite of Initiation.* London: Wisdom Publications, 1985.

Hopkins, Jeffrey, and Lati Rinbochay (trans.). *Death, Intermediate State and Rebirth in Tibetan Buddhism.* Ithaca, N.Y.: Snow Lion Publications, 1980 (2nd Edition).

Kariyawasam, A. G. S. "Anuttarayoga-Tantra," *Encyclopedia of Buddhism,* ed. G. P. Malalasekera. Colombo: Government of Ceylon, 1961.

Kiyota, Minoru. *Tantric Concept of Bodhicitta.* Madison: University of Wisconsin South Asia Center, 1982.

Lati Rinbochay. *Mind in Tibetan Buddhism.* (Elizabeth Napper, trans. and intro.). Ithaca: Snow Lion, 1980.

Lati Rinbochay and Hopkins, Jeffrey. *Death, Intermediate State, and Rebirth in Tibetan Buddhism.* Ithaca, N.Y.: Snow Lion Publications, 1980.

Lessing, Ferdinand D., and Wayman, Alex (trans.). *Mkhas Grub Rje's Fundamentals of the Buddhist Tantras.* The Hague: Mouton, 1968.

Lopez, Donald S. "Approaching the Numinous: Rudolph Otto and Tibetan Tantra", *Philosophy East and West* 29, No. 4 (October, 1979) pp. 467-476.

———. *The Tantric Difference.* M.A. Thesis, University of Virginia, 1978.

Mullin, Glenn (trans). *Selected Works of the Dalai Lama I: Bridging the Sutras and Tantras:* Ithaca, N.Y.: Snow Lion Publications, 1985.

Muses, C. A., and Chang. *Esoteric Teachings of the Tibetan Tantra.* Switzerland: Falcon's Wing Press, 1961.

Nalanda Translation Committee. *The Life of Marpa the Translator.* Boulder: Prajna Press, 1982.

Odin, Steven. *Process Metaphysics and Hua-yen Buddhism.* Albany: State University of New York Press, 1982.

———. "Fantasy Variation and the Horizon of Openness — A Phenomenological Interpretation of Tantric Buddhist Enlightenment," *International Philosophical Quarterly,* 1981, v. 29, no. 4, pp. 419-435.

Pott, P. H. *Yoga and Tantra.* The Hague: M. Nijhoff, 1966.

Rao, Saligrama Krishna Ramachandra. *Tibetan Tantrik Tradition.* New Delhi: Arnold-Heinemann, 1977.

Reigle, David. *The Books of Kiu-te.* San Diego: Wizards Bookshelf, 1983.

Sādhanamāla. (ed. Benoytosh Bhattacharya). Gaekwad's Oriental Series #41. Baroda: Oriental Institute, 1928.

Saunders, E. Dale. "Some Tantric Techniques," in *Studies of Esoteric Buddhism and Tantrism.* Koya San: Koya San University, 1965, pp. 167-177.

sGam-po-pa (sgam po pa, 1079-1153). *The Jewel Ornament of Liberation* (trans. H. V. Guenther). London: Rider, 1959.

Snellgrove, David L. *The Hevajra Tantra*. (2 vols.) Oxford University Press, 1959.

———. *Buddhist Himalaya: Travels and Studies in Quest of the Origins and Nature of Tibetan Religion*. New York: Philosophical Library, 1957.

Sopa, Geshe Lhundup. "An Excursus on the Subtle Body in Tantric Buddhism (Notes Contextualizing the *Kālacakra*)", *Journal of the International Association of Buddhist Studies*, Vol. 6, No. 2.

Sopa, Geshe Lhundup, and Jeffrey Hopkins. *Practice and Theory of Tibetan Buddhism*. New York: Grove Press, 1976.

Steinkellner, Ernst. "Remarks on Tantristic Hermeneutics," *Bibliotheca Orientalis Hungarica* XXIII, ed. Louis Ligeti. Budapest: Akademiai Kiado, 1978.

Thurman, Robert A. F. "Confrontation and Interior Realization in Indo-Tibetan Buddhist Traditions," *The Other Side of God* (ed. Peter Berger). New York: Anchor Press, 1981, pp. 208-250.

———. (trans., ed.). *Life and Teaching of Tsong Khapa*. Dharmsala: Library of Tibetan Works and Archives, 1982.

Tsong-ka-pa. *Life and Teaching of Tsong Khapa* (trans., ed. Robert A. F. Thurman). Dharmsala: Library of Tibetan Works and Archives, 1982.

———. *Tantra in Tibet*. London: George Allen and Unwin, 1977.

———. *Yoga of Tibet*. London: George Allen and Unwin, 1981.

Tsuda, Shinichi. *Saṃvarodayatāntra*. Tokyo: Hokuseido Press, 1974.

Tucci, Giuseppe. *The Religions of Tibet*. Berkeley: University of California Press, 1970.

———. *Theory and Practice of the Mandala*. London: Rider & Co., 1961.

———. *Tibetan Painted Scrolls*. Rome: Libreria dello Stato, 1949.

———. "Some Glosses upon the *Guhyasamāja,*," *Melanges Chinois et Bouddhiques* III, pp. 339-53.

Waddell, L. A. *The Buddhism of Tibet or Lamaism*. Cambridge: W. Heffer & Sons, 1895.

Wangyal, Geshe. *The Door of Liberation*. New York: Lotsawa, 1978.

Warder, Anthony Kennedy. *Indian Buddhism*, 2nd ed. Delhi:

Motilal Banarsidass, 1980.

Wayman, Alex. *Yoga of the Guhyasamājatantra*. New Delhi: Motilal Banarsidass, 1977.

————. *The Buddhist Tantras; Light on Indo-Tibetan Esotericism.* New York: Samuel Weiser, 1973.

Wayman, Alex, and Lessing, Ferdinand D. (trans.). *Mkhas Grub Rje's Fundamentals of the Buddhist Tantras.* The Hague: Mouton, 1968.

Willis, Janice Dean. *The Diamond Light of the Eastern Dawn.* New York: Simon and Schuster, 1972.

Winternitz, M. "Notes on the *Guhyasamāja-Tantra* and the Age of the Tantras," *Indian Historical Quarterly* IX/1, 1933, pp. 1-10.

Wylie, Turrell. "A Standard System of Tibetan Transcription," *Harvard Journal of Asiatic Studies*, Vol. 22, 1959, pp. 261-67.

Notes

(See the bibliography for complete publication data of works cited in notes).

1. Turrell Wylie, "A Standard System of Tibetan Transcription", *Harvard Journal of Asiatic Studies*, Vol. 22, 1959, pp. 261-67.

2. *rnal 'byor bla na med pa'i rgyud/anuttarayogatantra*, literally "unsurpassed" or "unexcelled" yoga tantra.

3. The other three sets of tantras are Action Tantra (*bya rgyud, kriyātantra*), Performance Tantra (*spyod rgyud, caryātantra*), and Yoga Tantra (*rnal 'byor rgyud, yogatantra*). The four sets of tantras are said to be differentiated by way of their specially intended trainees' varying abilities to use in the path four forms of desire: looking, laughing, holding hands or embracing, and sexual union. Only those able to use sexual union in the path are fit to be the specially intended trainees of Highest Yoga Tantra. The intended trainees are also differentiated by their ability to combine external activities and meditative stabilization (Tsong-kha-pa, *Tantra in Tibet*, pp. 162-3, and Dalai Lama's introduction, p.75. Also, see Jeffrey Hopkins, introduction to Tenzin Gyatso, Dalai Lama XIV, *The Kālachakra Tantra: Rite of Initiation*, pp. 30-38).

4. *Tāranātha's History of Buddhism in India*, trans. by Lama Chimpa and Alaka Chattopadhyaya, edited by Debiprasad Chattopadyaya, p. 343. Also, see A.K. Warder, *Indian Buddhism*, 2nd

ed., pp. 488-9, 491.

5. For instance, Jam-yang-shay-ba calls it the "King of Tan-tras" (Jam-yang-shay-ba, *Great Exposition of Tenets, cha* 54b.5). Almost two-thirds of the *Illumination of the Texts of Tantra* is devoted to Highest Yoga Tantra, and for that portion Nga-wang-bel-den apparently relied mainly on Yang-jen-ga-way-lo-drö's (*dbyangs can dga' ba'i blo gros,* also known as A-gya Yong-dzin [*a kya yongs 'dzin,* eighteenth century]) *Presentation of the Grounds and Paths of Mantra According to the Superior Nāgārjuna's Inter-pretation of the Glorious Guhyasamāja, A Good Explanation Serving as a Port for the Fortunate.* The *Guhyasamāja Tantra* is taken as the "general system" of Highest Yoga Tantra, the model in terms of which other tantras may be understood.

6. See the bibliography for complete citations.

7. For biographical information, see Lokesh Chandra, *Mater-ials for a History of Tibetan Literature,* Part Two, pp. 10-13, 282-284.

8. Jam-bel-shen-pen, as head of the Ge-luk-ba order, is called the "Throne-holder of Gan-den" (*dga' ltan khri pa*) to signify that he is the bearer of the lineage originating with Dzong-ka-ba, the founder of the Ge-luk-ba order, who founded Gan-den (*dga' ltan*) Monastery as the first monastery of his new order. Tri Rin-bo-chay is a Kam-ba (*khams pa*) who, as it happens, received his Ge-shay (*dge bshes*) degree at Gan-den Monastery in Tibet, be-coming abbot of the Tantric College of Lower Hla-sa after it was re-established in India and becoming head of the Ge-luk-ba order in 1984.

The Tantric College of Lower Hla-sa and the Tantric College of Upper Hla-sa (*rgyud sdod grwa tshang*) were the two principal centers of tantric education for the Ge-luk-ba order. Often, one entered the tantric colleges only after the completion of one's other monastic studies, which culminate in the Ge-shay degree, an indication of the Ge-luk-bas's genuine concern that one have a proper basis of monastic discipline, training in theory, and prac-tice of sutra Buddhism prior to embarking on tantric practice. The two tantric colleges have been re-established by Tibetan refugees in India.

9. See Bibliography under Yang-jen-ga-way-lo-drö for com-plete citation.

10. For instance, see works by Bharati, Beyer, Tucci, and

Govinda in the Bibliography.

11. See Agehananda Bharati, *The Tantric Tradition*, pp. 303-336, for an extensive, partially annotated bibliography. He writes: "The excellent work done by a few scholars who braved potential and actual criticism, and who dealt with tantric material ... appears like a drop in the ocean; an ocean that contains much redundant water, let it be said ..." (p.10). Also, there is a helpful bibliography including translations, editions, and other works, in David Riegle, *The Books of Kiu-te*, pp. 53-68. Among the few tantras that have been translated into Western languages are the *Hevajra, Chakrasaṃvara, Chaṇḍamahāroṣhaṇa*, portions of the *Saṃvarodaya* and *Guhyasamāja*, and fragments of others. In addition to the root tantras themselves, there is a vast collection of commentatorial literature that is virtually untouched. Very few studies have been done on the living tradition of Buddhist tantra (there are descriptions of rituals by Lessing, Snellgrove, Wayman, and a few others). One notable exception is Stephan Beyer's *The Cult of Tāra*, a fascinating and thorough exploration of the practice and theory of tantras of the Action Tantra (*kriyātantra*) class.

12. Tri Rin-bo-chay said that according to one text, teaching tantra without pure motivation would result in death within six months and birth in a hell (June 24, 1980).

13. A recent publication by Geshe Kelsang Gyatso, a Ge-luk-ba teacher well-versed in both sutra and tantra (Geshe Kelsang Gyatso, *Clear Light of Bliss*. London: Wisdom Publications, 1982, 254 pp.), is a general and moderately detailed commentary on Highest Yoga Tantra drawn from many sources and clearly indicates a trend toward greater openness concerning even Highest Yoga Tantra. There are a number of differences between Geshe Gyatso's commentary and Nga-wang-bel-den's presentation of Highest Yoga Tantra, mainly because the latter is based on the *Guhyasamāja Tantra* whereas Geshe Gyatso uses the *Heruka Tantra (Chakrasaṃvara)* for illustration.

14. The deities of tantric Buddhism are considered to be some of the infinite variety of forms taken by Buddhas and Bodhisattvas to teach sentient beings or to be of use to them in other ways.

15. According to Tri Rin-bo-chay, tantras are of two types, those that are the means of expression and those that are the objects of expression. The tantras that are the means of express-

ion are the books or spoken words of tantra, and the tantras that are the objects of expression are comprised of three tantras: the fruit tantra, Buddhahood; the path tantra, the graded path of tantric practice; and the natural or causal tantra, the natural causes in sentient beings' mental continuums that make it possible for them to become Buddhas (June 26, 1980). The basic meaning of tantra is "continuum" or "stream"; a book is a continuum of words, and the fruit, path, and natural tantras are also continuums.

16. "Vehicle" can also mean the destination to which one is going. The Hearer Vehicle and Solitary Realizer Vehicle, within the Low Vehicle, are vehicles for those seeking the ranks of Hearer and Solitary Realizer Foe Destroyers. (For an explanation of the translation of *shravaka* and *pratyekabuddha* as "Hearer" and "'Solitary Realizer'", respectively, see Jeffrey Hopkins, *Meditation on Emptiness*, n. 495, pp. 840-5.) Dzong-ka-ba explains that vehicles are posited either if there is a great difference of superiority or inferiority in the goal toward which they are progressing or if there are different stages of paths that give them a different character (Tsong-kha-pa, *Tantra in Tibet*, p.100).

17. Tsong-kha-pa, *Tantra in Tibet*, p. 106. He finds this etymology in the eighteenth chapter of the *Guhyasamāja Tantra*. According to Geshe Lhundup Sopa, in the tantric perspective the obstructions to liberation from cyclic existence are the conception of things as ordinary (rather than divine) and the obstructions to omniscience are those ordinary appearances themselves (Geshe Lhundup Sopa, "An Excursus on the Subtle Body in Tantric Buddhism", JIABS 6, #2, p. 52). This might suggest that the conception of ordinariness and the conception of inherent existence (the obstruction to liberation according to the sutra systems) are the same, as are the appearance of ordinariness and the appearance of inherent existence (the obstruction to omniscience according to the sutra systems).

18. The source for remarks on the three types of beings is Kensur Lekden (late abbot of the Tantric College of Lower Hla-sa), in *Compassion in Tibetan Buddhism*, (Ithaca, N.Y.: Snow Lion Publications, 1980), pp. 18-21.

19. Tsong-kha-pa, *Tantra in Tibet*, p. 104.

20. Chandrakīrti's *Commentary on (Nāgārjuna's) "Sixty Stanzas of Reasoning"* (*yuktiṣaṣṭikāvṛtti, rigs pa drug cu pa'i 'grel pa;* P

5265, Vol. 98), cited in Jeffrey Hopkins, *Meditation on Emptiness*, p. 200.

21. Sentient beings are drawn into a cyclic existence of death and rebirth due to ignorance. The subtlest form of ignorance, the actual "root" of cyclic existence, is identified by Ge-luk-bas (following their interpretation of the Middle Way Consequence School) as any consciousness conceiving that persons and other phenomena exist inherently, that is, from their own side, without depending on their parts, on causes, or on imputation by thought. Because sentient beings innately conceive phenomena to exist inherently, they easily generate desire, hatred, anger, and so forth, creating predispositions in the mind that have the capacity to mature into episodes or even lifetimes of future suffering.

22. The Form Body and the Truth Body have a relationship of being conceptually distinct within being an inseparable entity, or, technically, different isolates within one entity (*ngo bo gcig la ldog pa tha dad*). See Yang-jen-ga-way-lo-drö, *Presentation of the Grounds and Paths of Mantra*, 16b.3-.4.

23. Tenzin Gyatso, Dalai Lama XIV, in his introduction to Tsong-kha-pa, *Tantra in Tibet*, p. 50.

24. "Countless", according to former tantric abbot Kensur Lekden (1900-71) is a number followed by fifty-nine zeros; a great aeon consists of eighty intermediate eons (Jeffrey Hopkins in Tsong-kha-pa, *Yoga of Tibet*, p. 207).

25. Geshe Lhundup Sopa, "An Excursus on the Subtle Body in Tantric Buddhism", JIABS 6, #2, p. 50.

26. A yogi is said to gain vast merit by viewing "all physical movement, all verbal expression, and all thoughts and realizations as the seals, mantras and wisdom of a deity" (Tenzin Gyatso, Dalai Lama XIV, in his introduction to Tsong-kha-pa, *Yoga of Tibet*, p. 14).

Only Highest Yoga Tantra has this feature of great speed (although the three lower tantras do speed one's progress over the first two of the five graded paths, the paths of accumulation and preparation), and only humans of Jambudvīpa, the "southern continent" of four continents in the scheme of Buddhist cosmology, can attain Buddhahood in a single lifetime; gods (who are not immortal beings but rather are sentient beings with marvelous resources and lengthy lifespans) may attain Buddhahood within eight lifetimes (Yang-jen-ga-way-lo-drö, *Presentation of the*

Grounds and Paths of Mantra, 16a.2-.3). See Tsong-kha-pa, *Tantra in Tibet,* pp. 62-3.

Also, according to Tri-Rin-bo-chay, a principal way in which vast merit is quickly accumulated on the tantric path is the practice of visualizing the emanation of deities in a number equal to the number of sentient beings, imagining that thereby those sentient beings are set in Buddhahood itself. Incalculable merit is amassed through such tantric practices (February 9, 1981).

27. Tsong-kha-pa, *Tantra in Tibet,* p. 134.

28. Tenzin Gyatso, Dalai Lama XIV, in his introduction to Tsong-kha-pa, *Tantra in Tibet,* pp. 66, 69; and Tsong-kha-pa, *Tantra in Tibet,* p. 109.

29. Tsong-kha-pa, *Tantra in Tibet,* p. 65.

30. *Ocean of Feats, the Stage of Generation (bskyed rim dngos grub rgya mtsho),* quoted in the *Illumination of the Texts of Tantra,* 28.3-.5. It is also said that a practitioner of the Highest Yoga Tantra stage of generation nearly matches, in terms of realization of emptiness, a practitioner of sutra paths who has reached the eighth of the ten Bodhisattva grounds (Geshe Kelsang Gyatso, *Clear Light of Bliss,* p. 203). He explains that this is due to the fact that the Secret Mantra practitioner uses a much more subtle consciousness to realize emptiness than does the Perfection Vehicle practitioner. However, it is difficult to see why this is so for someone of the stage of generation, who has not yet manifested any of the subtler consciousnesses — the four "empties" — that are used to realize emptiness on the stage of completion.

31. This is a disputed topic; some scholars maintain that it would not contradict the Perfection Vehicle to say that the subject of which emptiness is being realized appears to the mind that realizes its emptiness.

32. Tri Rin-bo-chay, July 10, 1980.

33. P 6087, Vol. 153. Quoted in Sopa and Hopkins, *Practice and Theory of Tibetan Buddhism,* p. 21.

34. See Lati Rinbochay, commentary on Gendun Drub, Dalai Lama I, "The Two Yogic Stages of the Kalachakra Tantra" in *Selected Works of the Dalai Lama I: Bridging the Sutras and Tantras,* p. 151.

35. Tibetan traditions generally hold that the most realistic motivation for Bodhisattvas is to seek enlightenment as quickly as possible so that the welfare of others can be served in the most

effective manner, with the incomparable qualities of a Buddha. Although it is a commonplace in other interpretations of the Great Vehicle that Bodhisattvas seek to place all others in Buddhahood before becoming enlightened themselves, in at least some Tibetan traditions this is regarded merely as an exaggeration of the Bodhisattvas' concern for others, not as an exemplary strategy. See Jeffrey Hopkins in Tenzin Gyatso, Dalai Lama XIV, *The Kālachakra Tantra: Rite of Initiation*, pp. 14-15.

36. Tenzin Gyatso, Dalai Lama XIV, in his introduction to Tsong-kha-pa, *Tantra in Tibet*, p. 18. One Ge-luk-ba lama has written that "... those who practice Anuttarayoga Tantra must have renunciation, love and compassion one hundred thousand times stronger than that of the practitioner of Pāramitāyāna." (Ven. Gungbar Rinpoche, "Śrī Kālachakra", *Dreloma* No. 6 [1981], p. 14)

37. Quoted by Jeffrey Hopkins in Tsong-kha-pa, *Tantra in Tibet*, p. 207.

38. E.g., David Snellgrove, *The Hevajra Tantra*, p. 24.

39. Compare Stephen Batchelor, *Guide to the Bodhisattva's Way of Life*, (Dharmsala: Library of Tibetan Works and Archives, 1979), p. 131.

40. S.B. Dasgupta, *Introduction to Tantric Buddhism*, p. 72.

41. Jeffrey Hopkins in Tsong-kha-pa, *Tantra in Tibet*, p. 209.

42. This is the explanation of Tenzin Gyatso, Dalai Lama XIV, in his introduction to Tsong-kha-pa, *Tantra in Tibet*, p. 70, and in his introduction to Tsong-kha-pa, *Yoga of Tibet*, pp. 33-5.

43. Guiseppi Tucci, *The Religions of Tibet*, p. 51.

44. Tucci, *Theory and Practice of the Mandala*, p. 80.

45. Tsong-kha-pa, *Tantra in Tibet*, p. 161, quoting Viryavajra. A "wood-born" insect is thought to be one not born from an egg or womb, but just from the wood itself.

46. Mircea Eliade, *Patañjali and Yoga*, p. 179.

47. See Tenzin Gyatso, Dalai Lama XIV, introduction to Tsong-kha-pa, *Tantra in Tibet*, pp. 15-21.

48. See the *Illumination of the Texts of Tantra*, 20.3-.6. For a discussion of the various etymologies for *abhiṣeka* (*dbang*) see Jeffrey Hopkins in Tenzin Gyatso, Dalai Lama XIV, *The Kālachakra Tantra: Rite of Initiation*, pp. 66-68.

49. All the initiations of the three lower tantras are called vase initiations. The vase initiation is a rubric covering what are called

the five knowledge initiations — the water, crown, vajra, bell, and name initiations — and the vajra-master initiation (which is given only in tantras of the Yoga Tantra and Highest Yoga Tantra sets) as well as the appendages to all of those initiations. They are called vase initiations because in each, initiation is bestowed by way of a vase filled with water; either the vase is placed on the head, or water is poured on the head, or one drinks the water (Tri Rin-bo-chay, July 3, 1980).

50. For a discussion of many meanings of "mandala" drawn from Bu-dön, see Jeffrey Hopkins, introduction to Tenzin Gyatso, Dalai Lama XIV, *The Kālachakra Tantra: Rite of Initiation*, p. 75.

51. Tri Rin-bo-chay, July 3, 1980. He added that body mandalas are now used only in conjunction with the *Chakrasaṃvara Tantra*.

52. Tri Rin-bo-chay, July 3, 1980.

53. According to Tri Rin-bo-chay, actual trainees who can receive these initiations must have three qualifications: (1) they must have the pride and clear appearance of the deity, to the extent that they feel even when going to the store that they are the deity; (2) they must be able to hold back their emission of semen; and (3) they must be able immediately to turn a bliss consciousness into a consciousness that realizes emptiness (December 9, 1980).

54. The vagina mandala is not explained in Nga-wang-bel-den's text and was not discussed by Tri Rin-bo-chay; Kay-drup states only that the vagina mandala involves sexual union with a Knowledge Woman (Wayman and Lessing, trans., *Mkhas Grub Rje's Fundamentals of the Buddhist Tantras*, pp. 321-23).

55. See the discussion of the fourth initiation in the section on clear light, pp. 108-9.

56. The source for this paragraph is Tri Rin-bo-chay, July 3, 1980.

57. See the *Illumination of the Texts of Tantra*, 20.7-21.4.

58. A.G.S. Kariyawasam, in his article on "Anuttarayoga-Tantra" in the *Encyclopedia of Buddhism*, maintains that a tantri-ka of the Highest Yoga Tantra class needs and has no restrictions because he has already reached a level where his actions yield no result. That would imply that in order to be a practitioner of Highest Yoga Tantra, one would already have to be a Foe Des-

troyer (*dgra bcom pa, arhan*), one who has destroyed (*bcom pa*) all the foes (*dgra*), that is, the afflictions of desire, hatred, ignorance, and all of their seeds. Only those of at least the rank of Foe Destroyer have completely eradicated the conception of true existence; they alone perform actions that, without the motivation of ignorance or the afflictions based on ignorance, are without karmic consequences. Kariyawasam is clearly mistaken, because there is no tradition that says that one has to become a Foe Destroyer before one can practice tantra. A yogi of Highest Yoga Tantra who has not switched over from another path does not attain liberation from cyclic existence until the fourth level of the stage of completion.

59. See the *Illumination of the Texts of Tantra*, 77.6-78.3.

60. The *Illumination of the Texts of Tantra* says seven or sixteen lifetimes. Lati Rinbochay explains that if one guards the pledges and vows well and practices the two stages of Highest Yoga Tantra intently, one can gain enlightenment in one lifetime; if one guards the pledges and vows and practices as well as one can, one will attain enlightenment in seven lifetimes; and if one guards the pledges and vows but does not practice Highest Yoga Tantra, one will gain enlightenment in sixteen lifetimes (commentary on Gendun Drub, Dalai Lama I, *Selected Works of the Dalai Lama I: Bridging the Sutras and Tantras*, p. 157).

61. Nga-wang-bel-den's source is Dzong-ka-ba's *Explanation of (Ashvaghoṣha's) "Fifty Stanzas on the Guru"* (*bla ma lnga bcu pa'i rnam bshad*) and his *Explanation of the Root Infractions, Fruit Cluster of Feats* (*rtsa ltung gi rnam bshad dngos grub snye ma*).

62. Yang-jen-ga-way-lo-drö, *Presentation of the Grounds and Paths of Mantra*, 3b.2.

63. The *Illumination of the Texts of Tantra*, 21.4-.6. The discussion of the stage of generation is found on 21.4-28.6.

This definition is set forth by Paṇ-chen Lo-sang-chö-gyi-gyel-tsen (*paṇ chen blo bzang chos kyi rgyal mtshan*). Nga-wang-bel-den modifies it; he contends that not all yogas of the stage of generation mimic death, the intermediate state, and birth.

64. William Dwight Whitney, *Roots, Verb Forms, and Primary Derivatives of the Sanskrit Language* (Delhi: Motilal Banarsidass, n.d.), p. 132.

65. The latter part is taken from Tenzin Gyatso, Dalai Lama XIV, in his introduction to Tsong-kha-pa, *Yoga of Tibet*, p. 10.

66. Tri Rin-bo-chay, November 2, 1980.

67. The tantric systems assert that mind always rides on winds; therefore, even in the Formless Realm (*gzugs med khams, arūpyadhātu*), where beings are said to have no form aggregates, there is actually at least one subtle form, the very subtle wind in the indestructible drop (Geshe Lhundup Sopa, "An Excursus on the Subtle Body in Tantric Buddhism", JIABS 6, #2, n. 18, p. 61).

68. Tri Rin-bo-chay, April 24, 1981.

69. Lati Rinbochay and Jeffrey Hopkins, Death, Intermediate State, and Rebirth in Tibetan Buddhism, p. 14. See chart of six characteristics of each wind on p. 25 of Geshe Kelsang Gyatso, *Clear Light of Bliss* .

70. Geshe Kelsang Gyatso, *Clear Light of Bliss*, pp 24-27, has an extensive discussion of these winds.

71. Subtle winds operate at times of fainting, sneezing, and orgasm in the ordinary waking state, as well as at sleep, at death, and due to the practice of Highest Yoga Tantra.

72. In the sutra systems there are said to be 80,000 channels but in the tantric systems there are said to be only 72,000 (Tenzin Gyatso, Dalai Lama XIV, in "Tibetan Views on Dying" in *Kindness, Clarity, and Insight*, p. 172).

Also, according to Denma Locho Rinbochay, gods of the Desire Realm (*'dod khams, kāmadhātu*) and of the Form and Formless Realms have no channels or drops (oral commentary, June 22, 1978, translated by Jeffrey Hopkins). However, according to Geshe Kelsang Gyatso, tenth ground Bodhisattvas, who attain enlightenment in a Highest Pure Land, *do* have channels and drops even though they have the bodies of Form Realm gods (Geshe Kelsang Gyatso, *Clear Light of Bliss*, p. 217).

73. For the purposes of meditation, the central channel is visualized as blue, the right channel as red, and the left channel as white (Geshe Kelsang Gyatso, *Clear Light of Bliss*, p. 21).

74. According to Geshe Kelsang Gyatso, only four of the channel-wheels have knots, and of those, the knots are single except at the heart, where there is a triple knot (*Clear Light of Bliss*, p. 21).

75. Geshe Kelsang Gyatso identifies *ten* channel-wheels, adding the wheel of wind at the center of the forehead (hence, the upper opening of the central channel is placed between the eyebrows), the wheel of fire midway between the throat and heart, and

the jewel-wheel in the sexual organ near the tip (*Clear Light of Bliss*, p. 19). However, he says that the major channel wheels are six in number and are located at the crown, throat, heart, navel, "secret place", and sexual organ; knots occur only at the first four of these (p. 22).

76. Geshe Kelsang Gyatso, *Clear Light of Bliss*, p. 22.

77. The *Illumination of the Texts of Tantra*, 39.6-.7. However, even though the channel-knots prevent both the horizontal and vertical movement of winds, there appears to be some way that the winds can enter the central channel without loosening the channel-knots. This occurs in the level of verbal isolation when winds that have been dissolved in the heart enter the central channel without loosening the channel-knots above and below the indestructible drop in the central channel in the center of the heart. Even so, because those knots have not been loosened, the winds cannot move around, and an additional practice is required to loosen the knots. (See the *Illumination of the Texts of Tantra*, 41.6-42.2.)

78. Geshe Kelsang Gyatso, *Clear Light of Bliss*, p. 69.

79. Lati Rinbochay and Jeffrey Hopkins, *Death, Intermediate State, and Rebirth in Tibetan Buddhism*, p. 15.

80. For a detailed explanation of death, intermediate state, and rebirth, see Lati Rinbochay and Jeffrey Hopkins, *Death, Intermediate State, and Rebirth in Tibetan Buddhism*.

81. The mind of clear light of death is not the same as the actual clear light of the fourth level of the stage of completion, being just a "stoppage of gross dualistic appearance" (Lati Rinbochay and Jeffrey Hopkins, *Death, Intermediate State, and Rebirth in Tibetan Buddhism*, p. 48).

82. If conditions are not right for intermediate state beings to take rebirth within seven days, they experience a "small death" and take another intermediate state body. This can occur up to six times (Geshe Kelsang Gyatso, *Clear Light of Bliss*, p. 87, and Lati Rinbochay and Jeffrey Hopkins, *Death, Intermediate State, and Rebirth in Tibetan Buddhism*, p. 52).

83. With regard to the circle of protective deities, envisioning such around one is not the same as the generation of oneself as a deity and thus would not resemble birth. The same might be said of using an actual consort on the stage of generation. Tri Rin-bo-chay remarked that such practices could be viewed as preliminar-

ies or appendages to the stage of generation and thereby be excluded from it, but Nga-wang-bel-den clearly considers them to be yogas of the stage of generation (January 23, 1981). See the *Illumination of the Texts of Tantra*, 21.4-22.5.

84. For a description of the four yogas and six branches, see Dzong-ka-ba, *Great Exposition of Secret Mantra*, 686.2ff. For a description and chart of the four yogas, four branches, and six branches, see Stephan Beyer, *The Cult of Tārā*, pp. 114-18.

85. See the *Illumination of the Texts of Tantra*, 22.5-23.3.

86. Dzong-ka-ba, *Precious Sprout: a Final Analysis (mtha' gcod rin po che'i myu gu)*, cited in the *Illumination of the Texts of Tantra*, 23.5-.6.

87. The following description is just a small part of a much more extensive description given in Jeffrey Hopkins' introduction to Tenzin Gyatso, Dalai Lama XIV, *The Kālachakra Tantra: Rite of Initiation*, pp. 75-91.

88. According to two editions of the *Illumination of the Texts of Tantra*, (22.7-23.1 in the edition cited throughout this book) the supreme king of mandalas *and below (man chad)* go with the coarse stage of generation; this also agrees with Dzong-ka-ba (in a line immediately after the quotation above). Yang-jen-ga-way-lo-drö says the opposite, that the supreme king of mandalas *and above (yan chad)* go with the coarse stage (Yang-jen-ga-way-lo-drö, *Presentation of the Grounds and Paths of Mantra*, 3b.4), but it seems likely that this is a misprint or scribal error.

89. Dzong-ka-ba's *Great Exposition of Secret Mantra*, cited in the *Illumination of the Texts of Tantra*, 27.6-28.1.

90. See the *Illumination of the Texts of Tantra*, 23.3-24.4. According to Tri Rin-bo-chay, these designations are from the basic tantra (January 26, 1981). Also, see Stephan Beyer, *The Cult of Tārā*, pp. 71-75.

91. According to Tri Rin-bo-chay, the "period" (*yud dzam*) is one-thirtieth of a day, which would be 48 minutes (January 26, 1981).

92. Dzong-ka-ba, *Great Exposition of Secret Mantra (Collected Works wa)* 112a.6, P 6210, Vol. 161, 187.1.7-2.3), cited in Beyer, pp. 75-6.

93. Tri Rin-bo-chay, January 26, 1981.

94. Tri Rin-bo-chay, January 30, 1981.

95. Tri Rin-bo-chay, January 30, 1981. He added that there

are, prior to this, meditations in which one visualizes a subtle drop at the upper or lower openings of the central channel for the purpose of making meditation stable but those are not cases of visualizing an entire mandala in a drop. For instance, if one needs to avoid laxity in the meditation, one meditates on a sun disc on which there would be a subtle drop or hand symbol, visualized at the upper point of the central channel, between the eyebrows; if one needs to overcome excitement, the disc with its drop or hand symbol would be visualized at the lower opening of the central channel.

96. According to an Am-do (*a mdo*) lama's condensation of Dzong-ka-ba's *Great Exposition of Secret Mantra*, one attains this level upon getting mastery over the internal four elements of fire, earth, wind, and water (Tri Rin-bo-chay, January 30, 1981).

97. For this section, see the *Illumination of the Texts of Tantra,* 25.1-26.6.

98. Tri Rin-bo-chay, January 30, 1981.

99. See Jeffrey Hopkins, *Meditation on Emptiness,* pp. 67-109 for an extensive discussion of calm abiding and special insight.

100. Since, in tantra, one may realize emptiness even while appearing to the mind as a deity, it is perhaps not surprising that a union of calm abiding and special insight realizing emptiness could be achieved even while one was not at all involved with ultimate analysis — the search for an inherently existent subject — which sutra yogis employ to attain such a union.

101. Dzong-ka-ba, *Middling Exposition of Special Insight (lhag mthong 'bring),* Hopkins translation, p. 134, Thurman translation in *Life and Teaching of Tsongkhapa,* p. 176.

102. Tri Rin-bo-chay said that according to many books, stability is attained when one can stay on the object without laxity and excitement for at least four hours (February 9, 1981).

103. Tri Rin-bo-chay, February 9, 1981.

104. For an explanation of divine pride, see the *Illumination of the Texts of Tantra,* 24.4-25.5. Tri Rin-bo-chay explained that eventually, divine pride includes the thought that one is *all* the deities and even the inestimable mansion in which they live (January 26 and 30, 1981). Some persons fear imagining themselves in divine form, and this has led some scholars to say that Action Tantras are for such persons; however, such views are refuted by the Ge-luk-ba school (see Tenzin Gyatso, Dalai Lama

XIV, in his introduction to Tsong-kha-pa, *Tantra in Tibet*, pp.47, 58-9, and *Yoga of Tibet*, pp. 47-62).

105. Tenzin Gyatso, Dalai Lama XIV, in his introduction to Tsong-kha-pa, *Tantra in Tibet*, p. 64, and in his introduction to *Yoga of Tibet*, p. 12.

106. See the *Illumination of the Texts of Tantra*, 29.1-30.2. This is Dzong-ka-ba's opinion; Nga-wang-bel-den (30.1) may not wish to go so far, for he wonders if these should be merely counted as "types of realizers" (*rtog rigs*) of the stage of completion (and thus *neither* of the stage of completion nor of the stage of generation) or whether they should be counted as instances of the stage of completion in the continuum of someone on the stage of generation.

107. According to the *Illumination of the Texts of Tantra* (45.7-46.3), the use of an actual sexual consort on the stage of generation is very rare, and, if carried out incorrectly, will result in the practitioner's fall into a bad migration. On the other hand, it is said that sustaining a mind uniting bliss and the realization of emptiness on the stage of generation "ripens the roots of virtue for generating realizations on the stage of completion" (*rdzog rim gyi rtogs pa skye pa'i dge rtsa smrin*) and makes gathering winds by focusing on important places in the body, on the stage of completion, much easier.

108. Jeffrey Hopkins reported that this explanation is from Nga-wang-bel-den's *Word Commentary on (Jam-yang-shay-ba's) "Tenets"*. See Tsong-kha-pa, *Tantra in Tibet*, p. 240, n.72.

109. In the material Nga-wang-bel-den quotes, Dzong-ka-ba does not discuss the issue of the status of these persons because his point is simply that the paths they experience are to be posited as paths of the stage of completion.

110. The *Illumination of the Texts of Tantra*, 29.5.

111. Ibid., 28.8.

112. For instance, Chandrakīrti identifies five levels of Highest Yoga Tantra: the stage of generation, isolation, illusory body, actual clear light, and learner's union, according to Tri Rin-bo-chay, April 29, 1981.

Also, Nga-wang-bel-den notes (*Illumination of the Texts of Tantra*, 66.4-.6) that Jñānapāda's explanation of the *Guhyasamāja* system speaks of meditations on four drops or four joys. There, the four drops or joys are: (1) the indestructible drop at the heart;

(2) the secret drop at the "jewel" (the sexual organ); (3) the "drop of emanation" at the upper opening of the central channel; and (4) again, the indestructible drop at the heart, also called the "suchness drop". The first two are yogas of drops and the third is vajra repetition.

113. Geshe Kelsang Gyatso,, *Clear Light of Bliss,* p. 183, appears to consider physical isolation to be a yoga of the stage of generation.

114. Nāgārjuna enumerates five stages, the *pañcakrama:* vajra repetition (*vajrājapi*), purification of consciousness (*cittaviśuddhi*), blessing into magnificence (*svādhiṣṭhāna*), manifest enlightenment (*abhisaṃbodhi*), and union (*yuganaddha*). They can be correlated to the six yogas of this list as follows: lengthening vitality and exertion corresponds to vajra repetition; retention corresponds to purification of consciousness and blessing into magnificence; subsequent mindfulness corresponds to manifest enlightenment; and meditative stabilization corresponds to union. Withdrawal and concentration apparently come before any of the five stages of Nāgārjuna. See Alex Wayman, *Yoga of the Guhyasamājatantra,* pp. 163-173, esp. 173.

Dzong-ka-ba correlates the six yogas to the six levels of results as follows: withdrawal and concentration are included in the level of illusory body, lengthening vitality and exertion is the level of verbal isolation, retention is the level of clear light, and subsequent mindfulness and meditative stabilization are included in the level of union (P 5302, Vol. 158, 196.4, cited in Wayman, p. 167). The names of these practices are also found in other Indian yogis systems such as the *Yogasūtras* of Patañjali (Wayman notes that they are almost the same as the names in the *Maitri Upanishad*), but the Buddhist practices are very different.

115. The *Illumination of the Texts of Tantra,* 33.6-.7. Physical isolation is discussed on pp. 33.6-37.7.

116. See the *Illumination of the Texts of Tantra,* 31.3-.4.

117. The five aggregates are the aggregates of form, feelings, discriminations, compositional factors, and consciousness. The latter four are mental, the first, physical. The four constituents are earth, water, fire, and wind. The six sources are the objects of the six consciousnesses — eye, ear, nose, tongue, body, and mental — and the five objects are the objects of the five sense consciousnesses.

118. The meditation of physical isolation is not explicitly set forth in the *Illumination of the Texts of Tantra;* I have distinguished four phases in order to clarify the process further.

119. The description is consistently done in terms of a male body, but Tri Rin-bo-chay repeatedly stressed that women can practice tantra too. They may visualize themselves either as men or as women (altering the instructions where necessary), just as men can visualize themselves either as men or as women, as in the popular Vajrayogini practice.

120. In other tantras, concentration on a short (Sanskrit) letter *a* at the navel causes the Fierce Woman to be ignited (Geshe Kelsang Gyatso, *Clear Light of Bliss*, p. 29).

121. Tri Rin-bo-chay, April 20, 1981.

122. Geshe Kelsang Gyatso, *Clear Light of Bliss*, p. 57.

123. Lati Rinbochay, commentary on Gendun Drup's "Notes on Kalachakra" in *Bridging the Sutras and Tantras* (New Delhi: Tushita, 1981), p. 130.

124. Tri Rin-bo-chay, April 20, 1981.

125. Lati Rinbochay, and Jeffrey Hopkins, *Death, Intermediate State, and Rebirth in Tibetan Buddhism*, p. 15.

126. Tri Rin-bo-chay, April 3, 1981. The very subtle wind within the indestructible drop is also called indestructible because it is never separated from the very subtle mind.

127. Tri Rin-bo-chay, April 3, 1981.

128. Geshe Kelsang Gyatso, *Clear Light of Bliss*, p. 28.

129. The description of these four subtle minds is from Lati Rinbochay, and Jeffrey Hopkins, *Death, Intermediate State, and Rebirth in Tibetan Buddhism*, pp. 42-5. The etymology of the four subtle minds is from Dzong-ka-ba's *Lamp Thoroughly Illuminating (Nāgārjuna's) "The Five Stages"*, 225b. 1-3.

130. For a discussion of the characteristics of conceptual consciousnesses, see Lati Rinbochay, *Mind in Tibetan Buddhism*, and the introduction by Elizabeth Napper (Ithaca: Snow Lion, 1980), pp. 20-22, 28-31, 50-51.

131. A list of the eighty indicative conceptions may be found in Geshe Kelsang Gyatso, *Clear Light of Bliss*, pp. 82-5, and Lati Rinbochay and Jeffrey Hopkins, *Death, Intermediate State, and Rebirth in Tibetan Buddhism*, pp. 39-41. One of the eighty conceptions is the last gross mind to occur before death. One's lifelong habits and activities determine which conception will be the last

(Geshe Kelsang Gyatso, *Clear Light of Bliss*, p. 81). The nature of the last conception before death is very important because one's next rebirth is largely determined by that mind; if it is unwholesome, one will be born in a bad migration, whereas if it is virtuous, one will be born in a happy migration.

132. Geshe Kelsang Gyatso, *Clear Light of Bliss*, p. 73. According to Geshe Gyatso, the white and red drops cover the indestructible drop like a box; when they dissolve into the indestructible drop, one experiences the mind of black near-attainment. When they separate and continue their ascent and descent, respectively, one experiences the mind of clear light (*Clear Light of Bliss*, p. 86).

133. At the time of sleep, orgasm, and death, winds enter the central channel but one is generally in no position to make use of that occurence. It is not the case, then, that at those times one "comes close to opening the central channel" but cannot, as Thurman suggests in his contribution to *The Other Side of God*, p. 246 (see bibliography for complete citation).

134. Lati Rinbochay, and Jeffrey Hopkins, *Death, Intermediate State, and Rebirth in Tibetan Buddhism*, p. 47.

135. See the *Illumination of the Texts of Tantra*, 36.1-37.4.

136. Snellgrove, in his commentary on the *Hevajra Tantra*, identifies the four joys with four aspects of sexual pleasure. He says that the first joy comes from desire for sexual contact; the second from desire for even more sexual gratification; the third from the cessation of passion; and the fourth from the transcendence even of the third joy (*The Hevajra Tantra*, I, p. 134). His interpretation comes from the text of the tantra itself (II, p. 76) where the description is a little vague; it does not seem to have a similar application for *Guhyasamāja*.

Also, according to Geshe Kelsang Gyatso, there are four joys of the stage of generation in addition to four joys of the stage of completion. (*Clear Light of Bliss*, p. 99). The joys of the stage of generation, of course, are not caused by the entry, abiding, and dissolution of winds in the central channel.

137. According to Geshe Kelsang Gyatso, the fourth joy is generated when the drop reaches the tip of the sexual organ. This may, however, not rule out the experience of the fourth joy at the point where the white drop reaches the base of the spine, as in the other explanation.

138. The *Illumination of the Texts of Tantra*, 37.1-.3.

139. *Lamp Thoroughly Illuminating the Five Stages* (*gsal sgron*), cited in the *Illumination of the Texts of Tantra*, 70.1-.3.

140. Since emptiness is the nature of every phenomenon, and the "expression" of emptiness is a blissful appearance, it can be said that all phenomena actually are sealed with bliss and emptiness even if they appear to be ordinary (Tri Rin-bo-chay, April 17, 1981).

141. Tri Rin-bo-chay, April 17, 1981.

142. Ordinarily an explanation of *Guhyasamāja* would include 32 deities, but Nga-wang-bel-den explains that the latter twelve have not been mentioned here in the context of the twenty gross objects because they do not appear in the root text itself (*Illumination of the Texts of Tantra*, 36.6).

143. Tenzin Gyatso, Dalai Lama XIV, *Kindness, Clarity, and Insight*, p. 96.

144. Ibid., p. 97.

145. See Jeffrey Hopkins' introduction to Tenzin Gyatso, Dalai Lama XIV, *The Kālachakra Tantra: Rite of Initiation*, p. 110.

146. Ibid., p. 98.

147. Kenneth Ch'en, "Transformations in Buddhism in Tibet", *Philosophy East and West* 7 (January, 1958), p. 124.

148. Tenzin Gyatso, Dalai Lama XIV, *Kindness, Clarity, and Insight*, pp. 212-13.

149. The *Illumination of the Texts of Tantra*, 37.7-38.2. Verbal isolation is discussed on 37.7-43.5.

150. See the *Illumination of the Texts of Tantra*, 40.6-.7. The breath need not be associated only with those three syllables; alternatively, two syllables — HŪM and HOH — may be used, being associated respectively with inhalation and exhalation.

151. Tri Rin-bo-chay, May 1, 1981.

152. These three yogas concentrate on the heart, but in other Highest Yoga Tantra systems such as the six practices of Nāropa, the concentration is on the naval (Geshe Kelsang Gyatso, *Clear Light of Bliss*, p. 29).

153. Tri Rin-bo-chay, April 29, 1981.

154. Yang-jen-ga-way-lo-drö is, therefore, wrong to say that one passes to verbal isolation as the result of doing varjra repetition, the second yoga of the level of verbal isolation; see Nga-

wang-bel-den's refutation of his position in the *Illumination of the Texts of Tantra*, 42.6-43.7. Since the meditation on a mantra drop at the point of the heart is actually performed prior to the beginning of the level of verbal isolation, it would seem to belong at the end of the level of physical isolation. Mantra drop yoga has been included in the level of verbal isolation because of being the cause of verbal isolation, much as the meditation on a subtle drop containing a mandala of deities — a practice of the subtle stage of generation — came to be included in the level of physical isolation because of being the cause of physical isolation.

155. Tri Rin-bo-chay, April 29, 1981.

156. Lati Rinbochay, and Jeffrey Hopkins, *Death, Intermediate State, and Rebirth in Tibetan Buddhism*, p. 15, give a different account of the loosening of the channel-knots in the context of the process of death: as one dies, the channel-knots are loosened because the right and left channels become deflated as winds flow from them into the central channel. In tantric practice there is also a more forcible loosening of the knots; the *Illumination of the Texts of Tantra* likens the loosening of the channel-wheel knots to the process of opening the clogged hollow of a bamboo tube by ramming a long stick through it, an image of forcible rather than natural opening.

157. Tri Rin-bo-chay, May 1, 1981. It is apparently the case that one achieves different results from meditation on the secondary winds than when one meditates on the basic winds. For instance, the *Illumination of the Texts of Tantra* (41.2-.3) says that for the purpose of achieving various feats for the collection of merit, one practices verbal isolation on the four basic winds to achieve deeds of ferocity and pacification, whereas one practices verbal isolation on the secondary winds in order to achieve the five types of clairvoyance.

158. Nga-wang-bel-den (the *Illumination of the Texts of Tantra*, 41.3) says that the drop is at the tip of the "secret"; since it is said that the drop is "not emitted", this means the tip of the sexual organ.

159. Nga-wang-bel-den cites many opinions regarding the lowest point on the path where it is necessary to make use of an actual consort.

160. The *Illumination of the Texts of Tantra*, 43.5-.6. Mental isolation is discussed on 43.5-50.7.

161. Yáng-jen-ga-way-lo-drö, *Presentation of the Grounds and Paths of Mantra*, 8b.3; cited in Lati Rinbochay and Jeffrey Hopkins, *Death, Intermediate State, and Rebirth in Tibetan Buddhism,* p. 70.

162. Tri Rin-bo-chay, May 1, 1981. Geshe Kelsang Gyatso places these practices in the level of impure illusory body, as prerequisites for attaining the actual clear light (*Clear Light of Bliss*, pp. 204-6).

163. Tri Rin-bo-chay, May 1, 1981.

164. Geshe Kelsang Gyatso, *Clear Light of Bliss*, pp. 126-7.

165. See the *Illumination of the Texts of Tantra*, 70.6-73.2.

166. See Tsong-kha-pa, *Yoga of Tibet*, pp. 173-9, and Jeffrey Hopkins, "The Need for Common Feats" in Tsong-kha-pa, *Yoga of Tibet*, pp. 201, 208-9.

167. Tri Rin-bo-chay, June 26, 1980, and April 6, 1981.

168. That it is possible to have a mental isolation that is less than fully qualified is likened (48.1) to the fact that, as Maitreya's *Ornament for Clear Realization* (*mngon rtogs rgyan, abhisamāyalaṃkāra*) says, on the Mahayana path of preparation, practitioners, depending on their sharpness, may or may not have the signs of irreversibility (the signs that show that one is definite to become enlightened, namely, the disappearance of the discrimination of forms, etc., as truly existent). See Jam-yang-shay-ba's *Presentation of the Seventy Topics* (*dngos po brgyad don bdun cu'i rnam bzhag legs par bsha pa'i mi pham blo ma'i zhal lung*), *Collected Works*, Vol. 15 (Ngawang Gelek Demo, Delhi, 1973), 159.5-.6.

169. The *Illumination of the Texts of Tantra*, 51.1-51.3. Illusory body is discussed on 51.1-58.4.

170. Geshe Kelsang Gyatso, *Clear Light of Bliss*, pp. 97, 104.

171. Tri Rin-bo-chay, June 9, 1981, reported that according to some, because the impure illusory body has contaminated wind — wind produced by contaminated actions and afflictions — as its mount, it must dissolve before one can experience the mind of clear light.

172. This description of the illusory body's qualities is in Chandrakīrti, *Brilliant Lamp* (*sgron gsal*), cited in Geshe Kelsang Gyatso, *Clear Light of Bliss*, p. 188.

173. See debates and discussion in the *Illumination of the Texts of Tantra*, 52.5-54.7. According to Tri Rin-bo-chay (June 6, 1981), an illusory body is, like a Buddha's emanation, not bound

to any particular place; it can spontaneously arise inside or outside of the coarse body and move from there to other places. A Buddha can spontaneously emanate a body without having to travel to the place where it is to appear; likewise, he reasoned, the illusory body can suddenly appear anywhere, inside or outside of the body.

174. The very subtle body, wind, and mind are taught only in Highest Yoga Tantra, according to Jam-yang-shay-ba (Jam-yang-shay-ba, *Great Exposition of Tenets*, cha 54b. 5).

The identifications of the coarse, subtle, and very subtle are drawn from Lo-sang-gyel-tsen-seng-gay's (*blo bzang rgyal mtshan seng ge*, born 1757/8) *Presentation of the Stage of Completion of the Lone Hero, the Glorious Vajrabhairava, Cloud of Offerings Pleasing Mañjushri*, cited by Lati Rinbochay and Jeffrey Hopkins in *Death, Intermediate State, and Rebirth in Tibetan Buddhism*, pp. 31-2.

175. Tri Rin-bo-chay, April 11, 1981.

176. Tenzin Gyatso, Dalai Lama XIV, "Tibetan Views of Dying" in *Kindness, Clarity, and Insight*, p. 178.

177. See the *Illumination of the Texts of Tantra*, 73.5-.6. According to the Dalai Lama, since 1959 there have been at least ten cases among the Tibetan refugees in India of persons who have been able to remain, for at least two weeks without deterioration, in the mind of clear light that dawns at the time of death ("Tibetan Views on Dying" in *Kindness, Clarity, and Insight*, p. 178). Whether or not this means that all of those persons were able to attain enlightenment in place of the intermediate state was not said.

178. Tri Rin-bo-chay, May 4, 1981. This is sometimes called enlightenment *in* the intermediate state, even though one is not actually in the intermediate state, having risen in an illusory body instead.

179. See Herbert Guenther, *The Life and Teaching of Nāropa*, pp. 72-74, 197-201. According to his biography, the founder of the Ga-gyu order, Mar-ba (*lho brag mar pa chos kyi blo gros*, 1012-1096), became highly skilled in this practice and displayed it on several occasions, transferring his consciousness into the bodies of a pigeon, a lamb, a deer, and a yak (*The Life of Marpa the Translator*, trans. Nalanda Translation Committee, pp. 94-5, 146-55).

180. Geshe Kelsang Gyatso, *Clear Light of Bliss*, p. 126, says that the use of an Action Seal causes the winds to enter the central channel more forcefully, helping to loosen the knots at the heart channel-wheel.

It is interesting to note that Tripiṭakamāla, as reported by the Sa-gya scholar Bu-dön, holds, in contrast, that the very best trainees need neither a real nor imagined consort; that those of slightly less stature need only an imagined consort; and that the lowest of those capable of practicing Highest Yoga Tantra need a real consort (from *Condensed General Presentation of the Tantra Sets*, unpublished translation by Jeffrey Hopkins).

181. Tri Rin-bo-chay, June 6, 1981. He added that this is the reason why even in the lower tantras, a deity is imagined on an eight-petaled lotus; the eight petals of the lotus represent the eight petals of the heart channel-wheel when the illusory body rises there. For instance, in the mantra of Avalokiteshvara, OM MANI PADME HŪM, Avalokiteshvara is the jewel (MANI) that arises in the lotus (PADME), i.e., the deity that appears at the heart.

182. Tenzin Gyatso, Dalai Lama XIV, *Kindness, Clarity, and Insight*, p. 178. His Holiness adds that this is true for all sentient beings except for those to be reborn in the Formless Realm, who have no intermediate state.

183. According to Tri-Rin-bo-chay, this is a mistake, for a magician's illusion is a mere mental appearance, not wind (June 9, 1981).

184. According to Geshe Kelsang Gyatso, this example refers to the fact that a yogi who has attained an illusory body can manifest simulaneously in many forms, just as the reflection of the moon can appear simultaneously in many bodies of water (*Clear Light of Bliss*, p. 200).

185. Nga-wang-bel-den (the *Illumination of the Texts of Tantra*, 56.5) thinks that the sixth and tenth examples, likening the illusory body to an echo and to lightening, require modification when applied to an illusory body at Buddhahood, because at that time the illusory body does not abide in a fruitional body, but in an emanation body. Also, because emanation bodies may reside in coarse bodies, a Buddha's emanations may be anywhere, in anything. Hence, it is possible, said Tri-Rin-bo-chay, for people actually to meet with deities through statues, paintings, and other

objects (June 9, 1981).

186. Scent-eaters (*dri za, gandharva*) are beings with very subtle bodies who can live even inside of rocks and are able to subsist by using scents for food. They inhabit cities that seem to spring up out of nowhere and disappear suddenly. The *Illumination of the Texts of Tantra* compares the relationship of the scent-eaters and their city to the relationship between the illusory body's mandalas of the support and the supported. The mandala of the support is the mandala itself, whereas the mandala of the supported is the deities arrayed within the mandala. Like a city of scent-eaters, the mandala the yogi meditates on — of which, as a deity, he is a part — seems to arise and disappear suddenly (Geshe Kelsang Gyatso, *Clear Light of Bliss*, p. 200).

187. According to the Dalai Lama, a dream body can separate from the coarse body and go anywhere, even into deep space ("Tibetan Views on Dying" in *Kindness, Clarity, and Insight*, pp. 179-80).

188. The following identifications are from Tri-Rin-bo-chay, June 11, 1981.

189. In the following examples, the system of *Kālachakra* must be excepted, as it does not purify the intermediate state or have illusory bodies made of wind and mind (Geshe Lhundup Sopa, "An Excursus on the Subtle Body in Tantric Buddhism", JIABS 6, #2, p. 56).

190. The latter correlations are from Tenzin Gyatso, Dalai Lama XIV, *Kindness, Clarity, and Insight*, p. 97.

191. The *Illumination of the Texts of Tantra*, 58.4. Clear light is discussed on 58.4-62.3.

192. Tenzin Gyatso, Dalai Lama XIV, *Kindness, Clarity, and Insight*, p. 178.

193. Sarat Chandra Das, *A Tibetan-English Dictionary* (Calcutta: Bengal Secretariat Book Depot, 1902), p. 576.

194. Tri-Rin-bo-chay, April 3, 1981.

195. Geshe Kelsang Gyatso, *Clear Light of Bliss*, pp. 215-16.

196. Tri-Rin-bo-chay, June 12, 1981.

197. The *Illumination of the Texts of Tantra*, 62.3-.4. Learner's union is discussed on 62.3-64.6.

198. There is some controversy over the relationship of the mind of black near-attainment of the reverse process and the mind of clear light that precedes it. Kay-drup thinks that since

the afflictive obstructions are destroyed in the first moment of actual clear light, it would seem that the mind of clear light is an uninterrupted path of meditative equipoise and that the mind of black near-attainment that follows it is a path of release of meditative equipoise. (In meditative equipoise on emptiness, the uninterrupted path is the portion of meditative equipoise that actually destroys obstructions — either the afflictive obstructions or the obstructions to omniscience — and the path of release is the portion of meditative equipoise that follows the destruction of those obstructions.) He thinks that the verbal conventions of "uninterrupted path" and "path of release" are applicable because both consciousnesses directly realize emptiness, though the mode of apprehension of the mind of black near-attainment is looser than that of clear light. Those who disagree with him reply that the mind of black near-attainment, being dualistic, cannot possibly be a path of release; moreover, it is a coarser mind than the very subtle mind of clear light and thus is even a different type than it. Nga-wang-bel-den reserves his judgement, but Tri-Rin-bo-chay went along with Kay-drup, even going so far as to say that although a path of release is an exalted wisdom of meditative equipoise, it is not necessarily non-conceptual (June 18, 1981).

199. Geshe Kelsang Gyatso, *Clear Light of Bliss*, p. 211.

200. Geshe Kelsang Gyatso, *Clear Light of Bliss*, pp. 211-212.

201. Yang-jen-ga-way-lo-drö, *Presentation of the Grounds and Paths of Mantra*, .16b.1-.2.

202. In this paragraph and the two subsequent to it, information on the stage of generation is from Lati Rinbochay and Jeffrey Hopkins, *Death, Intermediate State, and Rebirth in Tibetan Buddhism*, pp. 69-70.

203. There are many other tantric systems in addition to these eight; for instance, there are six systems of *Chakrasamvara* alone. Bu-dön classifies some twenty-four tantric systems; see David Riegle, *Books of Kiu-te*, p. 20. One famous system not mentioned in Nga-wang-bel-den's list is that of the *Hevajra Tantra*, traditionally considered to be the original source for the practice of heat yoga (the Fierce Woman) found in many other tantras (Geshe Kelsang Gyatso, *Clear Light of Bliss*, pp. 34-5).

204. Although, with the exception of *Kālachakra*, the great tantric systems are quite similar, they have divergent emphases, generalized in the distinction between "father" and "mother"

tantras. The terms "father" and "mother" derive from the father-mother (*yab yum*) tantric iconography that depicts male and female deities in sexual union. The embracing figures symbolize the union of method and wisdom, the male deity representing method (great innate bliss) and the female deity representing wisdom (the mind of actual clear light realizing emptiness). Accordingly, Father tantras are those that emphasize method, and Mother tantras are those that emphasize wisdom, based on whether or not the tantra extensively teaches the illusory body (Father tantras) or clear light (Mother tantras). Tantras such as the *Guhyasamāja Tantra* and the *Yamāntaka Tantra* are considered Father tantras, whereas tantras such as the *Chakrasaṃvara Tantra* and *Kālachakra Tantra* are considered Mother tantras (Geshe Lhundup Sopa, "An Excursus on the Subtle Body in Tantric Buddhism", JIABS 6, #2, p. 54 and Geshe Kelsang Gyatso, *Clear Light of Bliss*, pp. 189-90). The classification of *Kālachakra* as a Mother tantra seems questionable because of the emphasis in *Kālachakra* on generating empty form bodies. Budön, in fact, sets it apart in a third category, shared by no other tantra, called "non-dual (*advaya*) tantras" (David Reigle, *Books of Kui-te*, p. 20). The Dalai Lama discusses both views in *The Kālachakra Tantra: Rite of Initiation*, pp. 159-60.

205. Dzong-ka-ba says that verbal isolation and mental isolation can be replaced by the Fierce Woman, and that this substitution occurs only in mother tantras (*Lamp Illuminating the Five Stages*, cited in the *Illumination of the Texts of Tantra*, 33.1-.2).

206. In mother tantras, it is called a "rainbow body of light" (Tenzin Gyatso, Dalai Lama XIV, in *The Kālachakra Tantra: Rite of Initiation*, p. 164).

207. For a description of the *Kālachakra* stage of generation, see the Dalai Lama and Jeffrey Hopkins, *The Kālachakra Tantra: Rite of Initiation* (London: Wisdom, 1985).

208. These differences are discussed in the *Illumination of the Texts of Tantra*, 79.1-81.4.

209. The Dalai Lama explains that the difference in channels, and so forth, between the *Guhyasamāja* and *Kālachakra* system stems from the fact that yogis have different types of bodies ("Union of the Old and New Translation Schools" in *Kindness, Clarity, and Insight*, p. 222). This would suggest that there are wide variances in the physical makeup of the subtle body, and

hence one needs to find a tantric practice for which one is physiologically suitable.

210. Apparently, five of the ten winds mentioned in *Kālachakra* are secondary winds, just as there are five secondary winds mentioned in verbal isolation in the *Guhyasamāja* stage of completion. Gendun Drub (Dalai Lama I) says that all ten winds can be subsumed under the five basic winds (*Selected Works of the Dalai Lama I: Bridging the Sutras and Tantras*, p. 165). He adds that there is a further difference — that the pervasive wind, in the *Kālachakra* system, mainly flows through the nostrils (p. 165). Ordinarily it is described as being responsible for the movement of the limbs and the vitalizing wind is involved with inhalation and exhalation. Some of the names are different; the ten winds mentioned in *Kālachakra* are: vitalizing, fire-accompanying, upward-moving, pervasive, serpent, turtle, chameleon, devadatta, *dhanaṃjaya*, and downward-voiding.

211. In the Middle Way Consequence School (*prāsaṅgika-mādhyamika*), the philosophical basis for tantra as explained by the Ge-luk-ba school (though the Mind-Only School [*cittamātra*] is also said to be acceptable), the basis for the infusing of karmic predispositions is the "mere I", the "I" which is merely imputed in dependence on the aggregates and which goes from life to life. In Highest Yoga Tantra, since the *final* basis of imputation of the mere I is the very subtle wind and mind, it is the very subtle wind and mind *in* the drops that is the basis for the deposition of the karmic predispositions.

212. The last two sentences are based on Geshe Lhundup Sopa, "An Excursus on the Subtle Body in Tantric Buddhism", JIABS 6, #2, p. 57.

213. Levels of the stage of completion are discussed in the *Illumination of the Texts of Tantra*, 81.4-90.2.

214. Nga-wang-bel-den quotes Dalai Lama I, Gendun Drub (*dge 'dun grub*), on the difference between the supreme immutable bliss of *Kālachakra* and the innate bliss of *Guhyasamāja;* the first Dalai Lama argues that there could be no difference between the two because otherwise at the end of the paths of other tantras one would be required to enter the path of *Kālachakra*. Rather, the supreme immutable bliss of *Kālachakra* is given a different name than the bliss mentioned in *Guhyasamāja* to denote its unique mode of production, namely, a different method for increasing

the drops. In the *Kālachakra* system it is necessary to rely on a Great Empty Form Seal in order to bring about empty form bodies. The Great Seal of Empty Form is a special type of consort who in some way (not specified in the text) surpasses an Action Seal. According to the *Kālachakra* system, if one did not use a Great Seal of Empty Form, the drops piling up and down in the central channel at the level of subsequent mindfulness and meditative stabilization would spread out at the channel-wheels instead of staying in the central channel.

215. Gendun Drub, Dalai Lama I, *Selected Works of the Dalai Lama I: Bridging the Sutras and Tantras*, pp. 177. For a more detailed description of the meditation, see pp. 172-175.

216. In general, the predispositions that produce wakefulness are located at the crown or forehead and navel.

217. According to the First Dalai Lama, Gendun Drub, the four night signs dawn as the result of stopping the coursing of four of the ten winds in four of the ten channel-branches coming from the heart, namely, those of the intermediate directions. The first four day signs are produced as a result of stopping four more winds from coursing through the four channels branching out in the cardinal directions. The final two day signs are generated by stopping the final two winds, which course through the channel-branches going up from and down from the heart, respectively (*Selected Works of the Dalai Lama I: Bridging the Sutras and Tantras*, p. 175-176).

218. According to the Dalai Lama, the signs dawn differently according to *Guhyasamāja* and *Kālachakra* systems because of the differences in the number of spokes or petals in the channel-wheels at the crown of the head and at the heart ("Tibetan Views on Dying" in *Kindness, Clarity, and Insight*, p. 174).

219. The day signs occur even at night "for superior persons" (the *Illumination of the Texts of Tantra*, 85.1). The explanations of *kālāgni* and *rāhu* are from Geshe Lhundup Sopa, "An Excursus on the Subtle Body in Tantric Buddhism", JIABS 6, #2, n. 50 (p.65). Serkang Rinpoche, in a talk in Madison, Wisconsin, in August, 1980, described the light of *kālāgni* as like star-light.

220. Gendun Drub, Dalai Lama I, adds that one visualizes that the sky is filled with the various signs and then that they dissolve into the empty form body of *Kālachakra* and his consort. When one's divine pride is fully developed, this level is complete

(Selected Works of the Dalai Lama I: Bridging the Sutras and Tantras, p. 177).

Also, although previously it was said that the right and left channels contained blood, semen, and so forth, they also contain winds in order for those substances to move about.

221. Paṇ-chen Sö-nam-drak-ba *(pan chen bsod nams grags pa,* 1478-1554), who wrote the textbooks for Lo-sel-ling *(blo gsal gling)* College of Dre-bung *('bras spung)* Monastic University, explains that although the meaning of *prāṇāyāma* in *Guhyasamāja* is vitality-lengthening — a life-lengthening wind — *prāṇāyāma* in *Kālachakra* means stopping the winds of the right and left channels and causing them to enter the central channel (from *General Presentation of the Tantra Sets, Captivating the Minds of the Fortunate/rgud sde spyi'i rnam par bzhag pa skal bzang gi yid 'phrog,* Dharmsala: Library of Tibetan Works and Archives, 1975, cited in Jeffrey Hopkins, supplement to Tsong-kha-pa, *Yoga of Tibet,* p. 265, n. 105).

222. The *Illumination of the Texts of Tantra* says nothing more about this practice; Geshe Kelsang Gyatso adds that the pot-possessing yoga, the vivid imagining of holding the winds of the lower part of the body in a pot-like configuration below the navel, is done to ignite the Fierce Woman (Geshe Kelsang Gyatso, *Clear Light of Bliss*, pp. 54-5). See Gendun Drub, Dalai Lama I, *Selected Works of the Dalai Lama I: Bridging the Sutras and Tantras*, pp. 179-80, for a more extensive explanation.

223. See the *Illumination of the Texts of Tantra*, 88.2-.4.

224. Tri Rin-bo-chay, July 2, 1981.

225. The text (87.1-.2) seems to indicate that the red drops may not begin to pile down until the white drops are piled up, but is somewhat ambiguous.

226. Nga-wang-bel-den says that at subsequent mindfulness one achieves a "non-imaginary" empty form body *(ma brtags pa'i stong gzugs,* 82.4-.5), but he is not certain that such has been "achieved in fact" *(dngos gnas la 'grub pa,* 89.6-.7). It appears that Kay-drup and others hold the position that the empty form body is achieved in fact whereas Dzong-ka-ba indicates that it is not achieved until all material aggregates are consumed. Also, Sopa (p. 58) indicates that the empty form achieved on this level is the cause of the empty form body of a Buddha on the next level.

227. Tri Rin-bo-chay, July 3, 1981. Dzong-ka-ba himself com-

pares the process to alchemy, the transformation of iron into gold (the *Great Exposition of Secret Mantra*, cited in the *Illumination of the Texts of Tantra*, 89.3-.6).

228. Tri Rin-bo-chay, July 2, 1981.

229. Geshe Lhundup Sopa, "An Excursus on the Subtle Body in Tantric Buddhism", JIABS 6, #2, p. 59.

230. The exclusion of enlightenment in the intermediate state is contrary not only to other tantric systems such as *Guhyasamāja*, but is contrary to the tenets of the Low Vehicle and Great Vehicle as set forth, respectively, in Vasubandhu's *Treasury of Manifest Phenomena* (*chos mngon pa'i mdzod, abhidharmakośakārikā*) and Maitreya's *Ornament for Clear Realization* (*mngon rtogs rgyan, abhisamāyalaṃkāra*) (Geshe Lhundup Sopa, "An Excursus on the Subtle Body in Tantric Buddhism", JIABS 6, #2, p. 55).

231. However, Nga-wang-bel-den (the *Illumination of the Texts of Tantra*, 89.6-90.1) points out that perhaps the fundamental wind acts as the substantial cause of the empty form body, since the very subtle mind of clear light, mounted on the fundamental wind, is generated in the entity of supreme immutable bliss. Therefore, the fundamental wind would be present at the time of an empty form body. He notes that there is no clear source saying that the fundamental wind acts as the substantial cause of an empty form body, and takes no position himself.

232. See the *Illumination of the Texts of Tantra*, 66.2.

233. Geshe Lhundup Sopa, "An Excursus on the Subtle Body in Tantric Buddhism", JIABS 6, #2, n. 52, p. 65.

234. The *Illumination of the Texts of Tantra*, 86.5-.7, indicates that the path of preparation lasts through the 1799th drop, when the path of seeing occurs; 1800 drops later, the second ground, the Stainless, is generated. There is nothing particularly unusual in positing more than ten grounds, for there are systems in which eleven, thirteen, fourteen, fifteen, and sixteen grounds are posited (Yang-jen-ga-way-lo-drö, *Presentation of the Grounds and Paths of Mantra*, 17a.4-.5).

Index

Right channel, 44, 73, 75, 119, 124, 126
in the *Kālachakra* system, 119
Rudra, 50
rūpakāya, see Form Body

Sa-gya School (*sa skya pa*), 15
sādhana, see means of achievement
sámatha, see calm abiding
sambhogakāya, see Complete Enjoyment Body
saṃgha, see Spiritual Community
saṃsāra, see cyclic existence
Saṃvarodaya Tantra, 158 (n. 11)
Scent-eaters, 101
Seal, 60, 88, 89, 91, 126, 127
See also Action Seal, Wisdom Seal, Great Seal of Empty Form
Secondary ill-deeds, five, 37
Secrecy, pledge of, 37
Secret Mantra Vehicle, 21, 23, 24, 25, 26, 31, 57
trainees of, 23
Secret place, 76
Seed syllable, mantra, 114
Seeing, path of, 42, 132, 133
Selflessness, 51, 58
of persons, 23
Semen, 119, 120, 121
Sense-powers, 59
See also eye-sense-power
Senses, doors of, 45, 124, 125
Sexual desire, 30, 33, 46, 172
Sexual union, 121, 122, 129, 179
See also absorption
Shākyamuni Buddha, 24, 92, 99, 107, 108, 109
Shāntideva, 31
Shay (*shad*), 86
Signs
day, 124, 125, 126
night, 124, 125, 126
Signs accompanying dissolution of winds, 73
Skull, 82
Sleep, 73, 76, 96, 102, 103, 104, 105, 106, 120, 121, 122, 172

Small capacity, beings of, 22
Smoke, appearance like, 74, 125, 130
Solitary Realizer Vehicle, 159
Sopa, Geshe Lhundup, 14, 159
Sound, pure mere, 121, 122
Sources, six, 70
Special insight, 56
See also calm abiding and special insight, union of
Speech, impure mistaken, 121, 122
Spiritual Community, 22
Spokes, channel-wheel, 44, 45, 119
Stage of completion, 27, 29, 34, 41, 46, 47, 51, 52, 53, 59, 60, 61, 66, 68, 70, 76, 80, 84, 87, 89, 91, 92, 94, 95, 106, 125, 129, 130, 133
definition of, 65
eight systems of, 117
levels of, 66, 170
See also physical isolation, verbal isolation, mental isolation, illusory body, clear light, union
Stage of generation, 27, 29, 34, 41, 46, 48, 49, 51, 52, 53, 55, 56, 57, 58, 59, 60, 65, 66, 68, 76, 79, 81, 91, 95, 110, 113, 114, 117, 129, 133, 169
coarse, 48, 49, 50
definition of, 41
prerequisites of, 29
subtle, 48, 49, 50, 59, 68, 71
Stage of imagination, 41
Subsequent mindfulness, 67, 123, 124, 126, 127, 133, 182
Suchness, 51, 52, 79
Suffering, 22, 30
Sun, 125
Sun disc, 168
Sunlight, appearance like, 74
Superiors, 23
Support and supported, deities of, 52
Support and supported, mandala